THE DARK FIELDS OF VENUS

THE DARK FIELDS OF VENUS

From a Doctor's Logbook

BASILE YANOVSKY, M.D.

A HELEN AND KURT WOLFF BOOK

HARCOURT BRACE JOVANOVICH, INC. • NEW YORK

PREFACE

In the fall of 1970 I found myself idle. The hospital where I was working had turned into an abortion mill, and I refused to take part in this destructive, although now legalized, activity.

While looking around for another job, I had an offer to work for the Health Department (Division: Venereal Diseases). In these city clinics I have come into close contact with an overwhelming number of patients, mostly of the younger generation and of both (if not three) sexes. The impact of this cross section of New York was such that I almost immediately reached for my old logbook of medical practice to enter there, as I used to, all that seemed significant to me. A selection from these entries (without their respective dates) I herewith offer to the reader.

The most dramatic test for syphilis, exposing the agent of the disease against a dark background under the microscope, is called the Dark Field. Hence the title of this book.

THE DARK FIELDS OF VENUS

1

"My boy friend went to a private doctor and was told that he has lymphogranuloma. That's a venereal disease, isn't it?"

"Yes, sort of."

"He told me to check it out."

"Well, I took your blood and a smear. You don't have gonorrhea, and next Tuesday I'll have the results of the syphilis test. As for lymphogranuloma venereum, we'll worry about that later. It evolves very slowly."

"How could he have gotten this disease? How do people get it? From sex?"

"Mostly."

Her eyes sparkled like a cat's; she was a slim, tall red-head—blue-eyed, very Irish.

"Now you know what to say to your boy friend!"

"Yes, I do." She gave me a conspiratorial smile.

"Since we are not sure, it would be nice of you to abstain until we get the results of your test. Anyway, Lent just started, didn't it?"

She answered with a young, joyful laugh, as if I had tried to say something really funny and succeeded.

2

She is a student at Columbia University. Twenty-two years old. Her boy friend called her the night before and told her that he has a rash on his penis. He is too shy to go to see a doctor, so he wants her to find out first. She went to Columbia's medical service but was referred from one place to another, until finally, at 6 P.M., she ended up at our clinic.

"Could he have contracted V.D. from someone else, or are you the only possible agent?" I asked.

"I doubt it; he's very shy. Last Friday we had intercourse. I was dead-tired and quite dry. He claims he had great difficulties entering me. Could that be why he developed the rash?"

3

"How old are you?"

"Seventeen."

"Do you understand French?"

"A little."

"*On est bête à dix-sept ans*," I said.

"I don't understand you."

"So your boy friend sent you because he had been here himself."

"That's correct."

"And do you have any complaints?"

"Actually I have no complaints, although at times I'm a little too wet."

"The test doesn't show gonorrhea. Are you on the pill?"

"Yes, I am."

"That might explain the wetness. Do you understand me?"

"Yes, I do." And suddenly she shot me a look of mature female understanding.

4

He couldn't believe he had it again.

"She just had an abortion a week ago. Maybe that's why I drip?"

"A week ago she had an abortion and you've started again already?"

"That's what I was telling her, too!"

He wouldn't believe me he was positive and went to the chief for confirmation and then to the lab for a new smear. He certainly knew his way around. But by the time he finally consented to the treatment it was too late. Patients have to be watched for twenty minutes after having received penicillin, and we stop giving injections thirty minutes before closing so as to be able to leave on time.

He got tetracycline capsules and was very disappointed.

"I'll complain. I know So-and-so, . . ." and here he mentioned a presumably very important man in the Health Department.

5

"My boy friend called and said he has it and for me to see a doctor right away."

"What does he have?"

"Clap."

"And you?"

"It burns a lot."

"Have you had V.D. before?"

"I had the same sort of thing a year ago."

She was a fair, healthy-looking girl of twenty-six. Not young, as patients at our clinics go.

"What is your accent—Scandinavian?"

"No, I'm English."

"Oh. And what are you doing in New York?"

"Visiting."

A few minutes later the lab report came in. It was positive. She took two injections, one in each solid buttock, without complaining.

"What is your profession?" I asked, trying to distract her.

"I'm a grammar-school teacher."

"Do you like teaching?"

"No."

She hiked up her tight blue jeans (no panties for her) and walked out.

6

A tiny woman, an eighteen-year-old Haitian ("no speak English"). She had come to New York pregnant, delivered, the baby died, and she was told in the hospital that she has syphilis.

"What does it mean?" she asked. "And how long will I be sick? My husband says he never had it."

"Is he here with you now?" We were speaking in French, and I found her French very difficult to understand.

"No, he's home."

She turned out to have gonorrhea as well. And since she was allergic to penicillin, we were obliged to initiate a lengthy treatment with tetracycline (up to 200 capsules).

We never hand out the entire amount, and she had to come once a week for her supply. Every time she came she insisted on seeing me. I had to explain, again and again, how she had to take the pills, and she would smile a very womanly, sisterly smile and say, "*Merci beaucoup, Monsieur le Docteur.*"

7

"Why can't you give me a shot today? Why do we have to wait for the blood test?" She certainly was impatient.

"Because I don't know whether you are sick or not."

"What difference does it make? If I'm sick, it will cure

me. If I'm not sick, no harm done." She seemed appalled by my stupidity. Altogether, she was not a very pleasant person.

"Wouldn't you like to know, twenty years from now, whether once upon a time you did have syphilis or not?" I asked.

"No, not really."

"What do you do in life?"

"I'm a buyer for a department store."

8

What I object to most in our homosexual patients is their asses. Why should they be so opulently dirty? It seems to me that people who use their rectum for business and/or pleasure should keep it relatively clean. Or at least when they visit a doctor . . .

Often they arrive in couples, like legal spouses, and the usual story is that "my friend told me he has it (or is now under treatment) and that I should see a doctor, too."

While waiting, they have a good time, joking, making fun of the doctors, the nurses, and the entire establishment. (The establishment, which no longer curtails them in their fucking habits, is their main target.)

If they have acquired syphilis—a very common disease amongst them—they are much less shocked than the heterosexuals. They take it as part of the game. Often one member of the couple is infantile or extremely immature, while the other is more sophisticated, cynical, and possessive.

The number of little lies they feel they have to tell is much greater (and much more naïve) than in the case of the regular male heterosexual victim. Many of them are barely twenty, and their eyes are pure, childlike, and absolutely untrustworthy. The over-all impression, in many instances, is of the actual presence of evil, of the knowledgeable serpent that generates such powerful attractions.

Usually they are cases for the Dark Field. If you scratch the sore and examine the exudate under the microscope, you may, if you are lucky, notice the *Spirochaeta* moving like a silver-gray corkscrew-snake against the dark background. (What you really see are the rays reflected from this microscopical beast and reproducing its image.) Homosexuals usually know about this test and submit willingly to it, although some of them are on the verge of collapse during the scraping.

Fewer lesbians come to the city health clinics: they go to a private doctor. They rarely contract gonorrhea; their disease is syphilis.

9

A plump, Irish-smiling girl. She showed up on March 17 and said, "I came to New York for the St. Patrick's Day parade, and I thought it would be a good opportunity to check on V.D. One never knows, does one? In my little town I can't go to a doctor for that."

"In your little town you have an opportunity to meet men and sleep with them, but you don't have enough privacy to go to a doctor?"

"Yes, if you want to put it that way . . . I have a discharge. I've had it for some time, but lately it has started to burn when I urinate."

"How old are you?"

"Twenty-two."

"Are you allergic to penicillin?"

"Not that I know of."

"What do you do?"

"I'm a writer."

"That's nice!"

Examination, tests, and treatment for gonorrhea she took

very courageously. When it was over I said, "Please, for one week no sex, no spices, no liquor."

"Oh." She seemed very disappointed. Then she said, "And how about pot?"

10

This blond girl, German- or Flemish-looking, very mature and womanly, although only nineteen, had walked out the day before, categorically refusing to lie down on the table and spread her legs for the examination. Today she returned; she had changed her mind.

"What's this? What's it for? What are you going to do?" she asked, watching every movement the nurse and I made. On the table, with her legs spread, she managed to bend in such a fashion as, almost, to be able to look into her own vagina together with me. The nurse had to force her head down into the right position. Then she started to scream. I told her to quiet down or leave, and finally succeeded in inserting the speculum.

And then she began to laugh. Homeric laughter: hilarious, triumphant, joyful. My first impression was that she was having a hysterical fit, but so innocent and radiant was her laughter that I had to change my mind. Later, when she was waiting on the bench for the result of the test, this laughter continued, gradually becoming softer and softer. Her outbursts, however, had alerted all the clerks (incidentally, mostly blacks). They could not resist its infectious quality and began to laugh with her.

I had the impression that this was how she behaved in bed, too.

11

He pointed to a small rash on his penis.

"Do you have reason to suspect a venereal disease?" I asked. It did not look very serious.

"Yes and no. You see, it was not a real sexual act: it was in the mouth; you know what I mean . . ."

"For you it was a real sexual act, wasn't it?"

"Well," he consented with a smile, as if appreciating a joke, "of course, if you put it that way."

I have noticed that, in New York, if people copulate in a special fashion, they do it not out of gourmandism but as a protection against disease or pregnancy.

12

"And remember, till we check again, at least for one week no women, no alcohol, no spicy foods. We don't want to stimulate the infection."

The boy looked at me with surprise.

"How about masturbation?" he asked very seriously, studying me with his cool blue eyes.

13

These meek, pale little neurotics usually come in with their belongings: an attaché case, a suitcase, huge cases for musical instruments (often filled with dirty laundry). They are dressed too warmly, and they are worried, very worried. The degree of worry is no criterion for their real condition:

they may have nothing, and they may have all the venereal diseases under the sun. They are neurotics!

If you tell such a fellow that he is perfectly all right, he doesn't believe it and continues to nag you. If you decide to give him penicillin, he will tell you that he is not sure whether he is allergic to it or not and that he wants to consult his family doctor (invariably the pediatrician) first. No psychoanalysis will help him. A good whore could save him, but where do you get a good whore these days, when they are all semiprofessionals or amateurs?

14

Periodically, old ladies from a geriatric welfare home are brought to us for blood tests.

They move slowly, if at all. Their arms and legs don't bend in the usual places, and they hate needles. Some are overly polite and grateful; some are drugged with tranquilizers and rude. But all are pitiful.

"Give me my tube!" screamed the old lady with the cruel blue eyes, chasing after the elderly Negro woman with whom she had come. It seemed to her that she had been robbed of this glass receptacle, which, a minute before, she had not even noticed and whose function she certainly did not know. But her companion, smiling an angelic smile, did not surrender the test tube. And both began to cry.

15

Next to the old crones sat eighteen-year-old girls: fresh, curious, joyful. Mostly Puerto Ricans, they all attended a school for beauticians; before graduating they had to have a blood test.

"No, Doctor, I can't look at it; my blood makes me nauseous."

"Hold your arm straight, please."

"Yes, yes, I will, but don't make me look. . . . Oh, is that all? I thought there would be much more to it!"

It reminded me of another patient, a young weekend bride, infected and abandoned by her husband, who told me in the same words about their first night in a motel: "I thought there would be much more to it."

16

A neighborhood community project has gathered up a dozen or so girls, all former drug addicts, in order to rehabilitate them. The girls are regularly sent to us for blood tests.

They have no veins: their veins have been "killed" by heroin injections. It is very trying to search for a patent vein when there are hardly any left. But the girls' co-operation is rewarding. First of all, they are not afraid of the puncture (unlike the men who come every two months to "check on V.D.," who obviously like fucking but cannot stand the sight of a needle). The addicts watch you search for a vein and direct you: "No, that one's no good; it's like a string. I never could get in there."

And if you have a skilled hand and succeed in drawing blood, they appreciate it: one artist applauding another.

"What are you doing in that project? Do they teach you something?"

"Don't worry, they keep us busy," one of the girls answered.

"Why do you sleep here?" I asked another who was dozing on a bench in the waiting room. "Don't you get enough sleep in your institution?"

"I don't sleep well there. In prison I slept much better."

Later, crossing the hall, I found two of the girls still hanging around.

"Why haven't you gone home?" I asked them.

They giggled. "We are waiting for our boy friends. They are getting examined on the other side," they explained.

17

"Oh, no, I can't look at my blood. . . ."

"Can you look at other people's blood?"

"Sure, that doesn't bother me."

"How ugly of you!"

"Why ugly?" She looked at me with surprise. No one in our presumably civilized society had ever pointed that out to her.

She is going to college and plans to become a teacher.

"What will you teach?"

"English," she said very soberly, busying herself with her things: with one hand she was still pressing the cotton to the oozing spot on her arm, at the same time clutching her coat and handbag and making for the door, because another patient was already entering.

18

"How old are you?"

"Seventeen."

"Really? I thought you were fourteen."

"Yes, everybody thinks so."

"From the scientific point of view there is nothing wrong with you."

"Then why do I have this discharge?"

"I don't know. Maybe some irritation. Maybe you overdo it. By the way, are you on the pill?"

"Yes, I went on it recently."

"That may cause a congestion. At your age I would look for other devices."

"Devices? I don't know what you mean. My father is outside. Could you talk to him, please?"

19

Two very young girls—teeny-boppers—were sitting on the floor in the hall. They wore mini-skirts, and their long hair covered their eyes, sheep-dog fashion.

Bending down to them, I asked, "Waiting for Godot?"

"No," they answered in unison, "we are waiting for our boy friends."

20

A group of Puerto Ricans came in: a beautiful, pregnant young woman, her two daughters, aged five and seven, and her smartly dressed blond niece. The niece had contracted gonorrhea from her boy friend and so the entire family, living together in a small apartment, appeared for a checkup.

"I want to make sure that no one else has this disease. I don't want my new baby to be born blind," the pregnant woman explained.

So we spread the legs of the little girls, too, and took smears.

Often couples come for a checkup together; not so much, it seems, for treatment as to find out who infected whom. This apparently is a source of constant conflict between them.

"You better tell him that I don't have it! He won't believe me!" a girl with a black eye implores.

And I tell him. (Sometimes I lie.)

22

She is a short, sturdy girl, blue-eyed, probably Jewish, twenty-two years old.

"It's a long story. Last summer, in Greece, I was raped, and ever since I've been worried about whether the man might have given me some disease."

"You've waited six months?"

"Well, you know how it is. First I didn't think of it, then I felt embarrassed, then I had the flu, and so on."

"What do you do in life?" I asked while waiting for the results.

"You mean, what's my occupation?"

"Yes. How do you make a living?"

"I'm an artist."

"What were you doing in Greece?"

"Tourist."

"Open to suggestions? You sort of asked for it?"

"Certainly not that man!"

"How did it happen?"

"I stopped at one of the foreign schools one evening; I had to make a telephone call, but the office was already closed. A kind of guard, a Frenchman, offered to let me use his phone. The moment I entered his quarters, he locked the door."

"Did you report him?"

"No. At first I was too shocked. I just wanted to run out of there as quickly as possible. And later they told me, better not, since there is no direct proof."

"How did you like Athens?"

"Well," she said, thinking hard, "I really don't know."

23

Yes, the junkies are a special breed; in a way a nice one.

They know what a needle is and are not afraid of it, and they co-operate intelligently. The trouble is that their veins are atrophied. It is hard work, and to be at such close quarters with them can be quite irritating, especially if they are dirty, with running eyes and noses, and laboriously breathing (many have asthma).

The majority of those who come to us claim that they are rehabilitated or on methadone, and, to judge from certain signs, this is true—except for their veins. The veins haven't yet got the message.

"Doctor, do you want me to find the vein?" a Negro, who used to be a boxer, said condescendingly.

"No."

After I had accomplished my job I said, "How often have I done that in my life? What do you think?"

He nodded approvingly but countered, "I've done it quite a few times, too."

A heavy, edematous black, with veins like strings and many scars on his arms and legs, sits across from me.

"Your veins are 'killed'?"

"Yes. I used to do it."

"And now?"

"Not any more. I'm in a methadone program. I come and speak to them. Sort of coaching the young and inexperienced."

"What do you think of methadone?"

"It's great. Now I'm holding down a job. Before I was detrimental to society."

He sounded like a propaganda pamphlet. He already belonged to the establishment.

Many of the girls from the community center are repelled by the idea of methadone.

"What's so great about changing one addiction for another? And for good—never to give it up again. For young people it doesn't make sense."

"No," says another, "I don't believe in such games. And it keeps you high, too."

"And what do you do at your community center?"

"We get group therapy."

But why do most of them look so sleepy and spineless, so absent?

24

Upon arrival our patients are given a number and have to wait. Later, one by one, they are called in by a clerk, whose vocation certainly is not writing and who has to take down their essential data and establish a chart. After that the patient goes back to the bench, to wait and wait and wait, until another clerk or a nurses' aide calls him or her for the blood test.

Sometimes a particularly plucky, impatient soul complains to the Central Office. As a result of such complaints, they may send us an additional doctor or nurse. That helps, but not where it is really needed: the bottleneck forms at the writing desk. Imagine a five-lane highway with only one tollgate; you may build a sixth lane on the highway—but that will not advance traffic one bit.

There is no air conditioning in most of our clinics. For emotional patients, after a massive dose of penicillin (2,400,000 units), this would be a necessity on a hot, humid summer day. (The administrators in the Central Office have air conditioning.)

Our elevator quite often and for no obvious reason stops running. But we have no way of knowing whether it is out of order or not; no sign can be posted, since there is no one responsible for posting one.

Having waited five minutes for the elevator, I walked up to the third floor to sign the doctors' attendance book. In the comfortable rooms women employees were reading and writing.

"Suppose you put up a notice that the elevator is out of order?" I said to one of them.

"I can't do that. It's not my responsibility."

"What's there to do? Give me a piece of paper. I'll write the note and hang it up."

"No," she said, "that I can't do. If you want to, you can speak to Miss G. She's in charge."

Finally they did hang up a sign: ELEVATOR NOT RUNNING. But they never took it down, so the situation is as confused as ever.

25

We have a special elite corps, a cohort of so-called investigators. They are our "detectives," who go after potential syphilitics and their contacts to make them come to our clinic.

These are youngsters with barely a college education and a month's training in detective procedures, but they like to think of themselves as social workers, psychotherapists, scientists, doctors.

Such young people could of course help the admitting clerk, for they certainly are literate. But they prefer to initiate every newly established syphilitic into the physiology and pathology as well as the sexual implications of his or her disease. Quite often I find a young investigator closeted in a small room, showing frightening, vividly colored pictures to a young patient, or a young female investigator enlightening a young male about the sores on his penis. On and off I have a feeling that the pleasure they derive from this activity is of a questionable nature.

"It's exciting," one girl investigator told me with a radiant smile. She was dressed in a floor-length gypsy costume, cut so low at the neck that it showed the better part of her breasts.

There is clearly a conflict between the investigators and the other employees of our clinics. "They try to run the show" is the general complaint.

26

They were locked in a small compartment: she, the investigator, supposedly instructing him, the patient, how to behave.

"Every time I've been with a woman it begins to drip again."

"You don't say." She looked with sympathy at his young, virile Spanish face.

My locker was in the same room. I had entered to change from my white gown into street clothes. And both, patient and investigator, were waiting for me to leave. I was intruding; they needed privacy.

Incidentally, we spend millions on penicillin and disposable materials, but to get a clean gown at least once a week, in a clinic where everything seems to be dripping, is all but impossible: "I don't take care of that. Ask Mrs. T. about it."

27

She is a music student: piano and composition. Likes Beethoven and Schumann, Chopin much less, but, above all, Bach. Her boy friend, also a musician, told her that he "got it." And she would like to make sure about herself.

"How old are you?"

"Twenty-eight."

"I can hardly believe it." She looked eighteen.

"Yes. I'm divorced and have two children."

"How do you think your boy friend got it?"

"I don't know. I'd like to know."

A little while later I told her that she had it, too.

"Have what?"

"Gonorrhea. For the result of the syphilis test you'll have to come back next week."

She hesitated and then said, "My girl friend came along with me. She'd like a checkup, too."

"You mean she slept with the same musician?"

"I don't know. I wonder."

There was nothing wrong with the girl friend. Since she claimed to be a virgin, I did not do the cervical smear. She volunteered, however, that she was on the pill: "Just in case. To be ready." And she smiled a dreamy smile.

28

She was sent by the court. A prostitute, when arrested, automatically goes through an examination; regardless of the

initial tests, she is classified G 90, t.e., epidemiologic gonorrhea, and given preventive treatment.

This one was a grossly overweight girl, who in five years
or so would be a monstrosity. For the time being, dark-eyed,
intelligent, and sensual, apparently a Mediterranean and with
some education, she was very attractive.

"Why do you do it?" I asked.

"I don't know."

She was circumspect and slow in her answers but did not
duck the issue.

"This is New York," I said. "An intelligent person can
make an honest living."

"I don't like to work. Especially not for peanuts. And you
have to sleep with the boss, anyway. I've been through that."

"Yes, I imagine so. Men must be sniffing around you all
the time."

She laughed, flattered.

A week or so later I was on the men's side, when she and
an escort walked in together and sat down on the bench. He
was an extremely good-looking man, a Mediterranean gigolo
type, but unshaven. She was dressed up and looked festive.
When she spotted me in the next room, she bent to her
man and said something. They both turned in my direction
and, smiling encouragingly, waved to me. My feeling was
that she had said to him, "There is that nice jerk from last
week I told you about."

29

"I just want a checkup."

"Any special reason?"

"No. I just want to check out on V.D."

"Anything happened lately?"

"Last Friday I was stone-drunk."

"And you slept with someone?"

"Yes, apparently. I was bombed."

While working on her: "What is your occupation?"

"Just wasting myself."

"Why don't you work?"

"There's no work now in New York."

"Did you finish school?"

"Yes, thank God, I had enough sense."

"What school? College or high school?"

"High school, of course."

After the report of the vaginal smear came back from the lab: "You do have gonorrhea."

"Is it bad?"

"We'll take care of you. Are you going to meet this fellow again?"

"What for?"

"It would be nice if you could get him to go and see a doctor, too."

"I might run into him around Penn Station."

"What are you doing at Penn Station?"

"That's where I usually hang out."

She was barely twenty, a semiprofessional, plump, unkempt, and confused.

30

A girl of eighteen.

"It worries me; I'd like to make sure."

"Did you take a chance with a stranger?"

"Not really. He's from my home town. But I'm worried."

"Do you have any discharge, any sores?"

"Only a little discharge."

"Are you on the pill?"

"No, I'm not."

"What kind of precautions do you take?"

any more of this nonsense." And to her surprise, I took her firmly by the elbow and escorted her to the door.

Later, another doctor told me proudly that he had succeeded in taking her blood. Whether he could have done so if I had not thrown her out of my room remained a moot question.

38

"Doctor, I think I have it."
"What's the story?"
"Yesterday morning I met a girl, and now I think I drip."
"Discharge? Burning?"
"Yes."
"How can you afford to fool around with a girl on a weekday morning?"
"She didn't ask much—only twenty dollars."
He was a well-dressed young Negro.

39

A middle-aged Jewish man with a worried look: "What's it all about, anyway? You pay them good money and then you have to take care of yourself. If I got it, I'll never touch one again. Just tell me, Doctor."
The answer was yes.

40

"I want to make sure. I'm living with a girl, but she goes with other men and I go with other women." Young, with a fine, silky beard, he looked like an early-Renaissance monk.

As it happened, he did not have it. I told him and added, "But one of these days you'll get it. If both of you go in different directions, why stay together? It doesn't make sense."

"How strange that you say that," he began, but I interrupted him.

"I'm sorry, perhaps it isn't a doctor's business to speak like that, but I can't help it."

"No. No. What you said is tremendous! If only other people would talk like that." And extending his arm, he suddenly shook my hand, giving me the beautiful smile of an early-Renaissance monk.

41

She had a little erosion, an ulcer, on the right vulva lip. While the bacteriologist was digging in with his needle (to get the juice onto the slide for the Dark Field), I watched her: a strong, healthy female whose only attraction lay in her youth.

"What precautions do you take?" I asked.

"I have a loop."

"The bleeding may come from the loop. Some people can't tolerate it."

"What do you mean 'tolerate'?"

"How long have you been wearing it?"

"Four years."

"My God, how come you've never taken it out?"

"I don't know."

"And this man who gave you syphilis—do you know him?"

"I know him."

42

The familiar story: her boy friend called to tell her that he has it. He thinks she gave it to him, and he doesn't want to see her any more.

Her first tests were negative.

"We must classify her G 90," said the nurse. That would call for a strong preventive dose of penicillin.

"Suppose this man wants to get rid of her and invented a pretext. Why should we believe him?" I asked the nurse, while the girl followed the discussion with great approval. I decided to let her go. In two weeks, after the results of the culture for gonorrhea were in, we would see our way better.

43

A thirty-four-year-old Hungarian woman, working as a maid in a cheap hotel, came in because her boy friend was receiving treatment for gonorrhea at our clinic. She looked older than her years, precociously worn, downtrodden; tired of life and of work, of the English language, which she cannot master, and of the men who pursue her in the narrow corridors of her obscure hotel.

Indeed, she did have gonorrhea.

"Doctor, my boy friend and I know who gave it to him. We would like to give you her name so you can stop her." She explained this to me with more hatred in her voice than dejection over her new sickness. And while getting dressed she took it up again.

"Doctor, what can I do about this woman? Tell me that."

She wanted justice or revenge, whichever you want to call it.

44

Two girl students, one after the other.

The first, black, sexy, very clean: all her essential organs kept in emergency readiness, shining like the guns of a practiced sniper.

The second, a white intellectual, apparently from a good background, unkempt, and really filthy around her genitals. "Do you sometimes take a douche?"

"No," she said, "what's it for?"

45

For the first time I had a lesbian couple. Both Puerto Rican, fortyish, one heavy, with huge breasts, the other lean and muscular. The lean one had officially come along as translator. It was the obese one who wanted to be checked for syphilis.

"Why do you suspect that you might have syphilis?" I asked through the translator. "Did you sleep with someone who might have it?"

"Yes," the answer came back.

"And who is this person? Can you locate him?"

"It's me," stated the translator. "But I was treated last February and don't need any advice."

46

He wanted a smear from his rectum. He started in a foggy fashion and took some time to indicate the place that worried him. I cast a glance there and noticed an abrasion.

"Does it hurt?"

"It did. It's better now."

We dug into this small ulcer for a Dark Field examination and a short while later the bacteriologist showed me two dangerously slim, beautifully slithering *Spirochaetae pallidae* under the microscope. Their fine, silvery, corkscrew silhouettes conveyed a truly ominous impression.

47

From time to time men from the merchant marine with old histories of V.D. are sent to us. We are unable to get coherent information from them since they speak Spanish or Greek or Portuguese but not a word of English.

The right thing would be to take a blood sample and wait a week for the results of the tests. But the shipping companies and the unions want immediate treatment. The ship is usually sailing within twenty-four hours, and they can't afford to have a cook or a steward with a possible case of acute syphilis on board.

So we give them a maximum dose of penicillin, even if we aren't sure they need it. Society needs it.

48

Sometimes a special kind of couple appears in our waiting room: two boys, one of them not only dressed as but virtually transformed into a woman. So gentle, so delicate is "she," so colorful and dainty the silky underwear, that I, too, become confused and call him her.

How they suffer when they have to show their private parts! A small penis, a small, soft nothing, all wrapped in powdered tissue. So much powder that while "she" unwraps, some is blown into my face. Only their voices they cannot transform. Often it is a particularly low masculine basso. (Or does it only seem so low by way of contrast?)

The impression is of a vicious monstrosity, a mad and cruel invention. These are transvestites. Quite a different breed from the regular homosexual couples who appear at my desk and meekly or aggressively proffer their asses.

49

"What makes you think you have it?" I asked the young lawyer.

"I met a girl on St. Patrick's Day, and after a couple of drinks we went to bed. You know how it is on St. Patrick's Day."

"Are you Irish?"

"No, I'm German."

"Is she Irish?"

"I wish she was, then I wouldn't have to worry so much. No, she's English."

After the examination I said, "You don't have gonorrhea. We call this nongonococci urethritis. It's an infection with banal microbes. It may be very annoying, but it's not V.D. At least that's how we classify it. I'll give you some capsules, and if they don't help you'll have to go to the urology department at a city hospital. They are supposed to take care of such things."

"Oh, thank you, Doctor, thank you very much, I'm so glad. . . ."

(When they've got it, they never thank the doctor. They feel gratitude only when the test is negative.)

He was already out in the hall when I yelled after him, "Maybe she wasn't English; maybe she was half Irish!"

It took the lawyer a good moment to grasp my joke. But he did finally, and grinned.

50

"As far as I know, I don't have any venereal disease."

"Well, you see, our investigators found out from a new syphilis case that you were his last contact. That makes you a suspect for syphilis."

"So now you are going to treat me, too? Can't you wait until the results of the test are available?"

His question was fully justified. But I answered, "According to our rules we can't wait. We have to classify you as S 90, which means epidemiological syphilis, and we give you your first shot of penicillin. The second you get only if your test is positive."

"And what if I blow up from the penicillin, if I collapse or stop breathing?"

"That would be too bad. But you said you are not allergic to penicillin."

"I said I don't know. I said I've never taken any."

"That's all the Health Department needs to know."

"What's going on, anyway? Are you the police?"

"No. But for the well-being of the many we must sacrifice the interest of the individual."

"The hell with you and your medicine," the cruel-mouthed, gray-haired man exclaimed. "Now I remember. My doctor told me I'm allergic to penicillin."

"That's different. Then you'll get pills. One hundred capsules of tetracycline."

"What? All at once?"

"No, you'll take twelve a day. We'll give you a supply."

"You make me laugh." And he walked out with his supply of pills.

51

A middle-aged black with a half-empty pint of whiskey in his hand was sitting on the bench, making a lot of noise. He laughed, cursed, coughed, and even tried to dance a jig between the benches.

"What is this nuisance doing here?" I asked the nurse.

"He's come with a friend and is waiting for him."

The friend, to my surprise, turned out to be a well-dressed, well-mannered white man of twenty-five. He had gonorrhea and accused his girl friend of having infected him. He had tried to bring her in, too, but a block from the clinic she had given him the slip.

I tried to process the young man quickly so as to get rid of the drunken black. The basis of their association I couldn't figure out. The older man was obviously protecting the younger one, and, judging by their totally disparate appearances, it had to be a metaphysical sort of patronage.

While I was doing my work, the drunkard continued to laugh, sing, pull funny faces, and to repeat my words and copy my gestures. Suddenly I realized what he was doing: he was trying hard to cheer us all up. . . .

52

He came in: red-bearded, slightly graying, tall, fiftyish, and still going strong. A Viking—but tanned by the tropical sun.

He thinks he has gonorrhea. He is very rushed, very busy. Just in from his island for a couple of days. Tomorrow he is going back, to the West Indies.

"Did you notice burning or a discharge from your rectum?"

"No. But my little friend has it."

The little friend was a very shy, very pretty black boy. Their tests showed no gonococci.

"I'm surprised," the Viking complained. "I could swear I have it. I know he has."

I repeated the tests on both; mistakes do happen. But the results were negative again.

"You have a urethritis, but it is not V.D.," I started listlessly. Twenty times a day I have to elaborate on this subject, and my patients never are able to grasp why, since they have an infection, I do not treat them. But the Viking understood. With grace he accepted the pills that I handed him.

I didn't get around to ask him his occupation. A couple of centuries ago he would have been a pirate or a searcher after buried pirate treasure. In our time he could be selling arms to some obscure Caribbean rebels. He had a penis proportionate to his build, and I could not imagine how it possibly could enter the shy boy's little opening.

53

"Perhaps you weren't sensible. Perhaps you didn't behave. You know, the shots alone don't cure."

"You mean no women, no spices, no liquor. I behaved. Last Friday I was at a party, and I really could have scored, but my conscience wouldn't let me."

"It's not a question only of scoring with women," I said. "It's a question of avoiding excitement, stimulation, erection."

"Oh." He was genuinely bewildered. "No one ever told me that. . . . But you can't always avoid an erection," he added very soberly. "You know, in the morning when you wake up and lie on your back."

"While you are under treatment, for a week or two, take a cold shower immediately after you wake up."
He laughed, surprised, but apparently approving my logic.

54

"What's your profession?"
"I'm an airline stewardess. I've never had clap before, but he claims he got it from me."
"For the moment, all your tests are negative. Come back in a week for the final results."
"I can't. Next Tuesday I'll be in New Delhi."
"Then come in two weeks."
"Would that be all right?"
"Yes, provided you behave meanwhile. No sex, you understand."
"Oh, I do. I'll behave. I don't really enjoy it," she said. Her Oriental face looked radiant, almost saintly.

55

A little blonde, fresh and juicy as an apricot.
"He told me I should see a doctor."
"Have you any symptoms?"
"What do you mean? I don't understand."
"Do you have a discharge? Any sores?"
"No, I don't think so. I have a little discharge. You know, the usual one."
"Are you on the pill?"
"No, I don't take any precautions."
"Oh. How come?"
"I do it so seldom. I'm a stranger in New York."
"What are you doing here?"

"I study drama. Acting."

"Do you like Beckett?"

"Who is that? I haven't been long in New York—I don't know all the names."

"But you do know your boy friend?"

"Not really well."

"Do you like him?"

"Who? My boy friend?" She reflected for a moment, fixing her round blue eyes on some imaginary object, and then, with the sigh of a woman who has just given birth, said, "Yes, I do."

56

"They sent me here from St. Mark's Clinic," she said belligerently, handing me a note. St. Mark's Clinic is run by idealistic people who don't have the proper (expensive) equipment; every now and then they send us a patient with suspicious sores for the Dark Field examination.

This girl had two such sores in the folds of her genitals. I asked for a Dark Field on each, but our bacteriologist, claiming that he was too busy, took the slides only from one. The result was negative. And yet I had the distinct impression that that was a syphilitic chancre. But we have no authority over our lab technicians.

57

"His serology is slightly positive, one to four," said the chief. "He denies any past history of syphilis."

"I wouldn't take any chances with this fellow. Order a full treatment," said the other doctor.

"You are ready to give a massive dose of penicillin on the

basis of one weakly positive test?" I tried to defend my patient. (There are many conditions and diseases besides syphilis that can produce a weak immunological reaction. People who have been cured of syphilis carry a "scar" in their blood; malaria and some other tropical diseases can give a false positive; heroin addicts, too, fool you.) "Let's at least repeat the blood test. What's the rush? He's lived for decades with this serology," I moved.

"No, I won't take any chances," the chief decided.

"Suppose it was the Duke of Windsor; would you also start treatment now?"

"What are you talking about?" said the chief, giving me a disgusted look.

58

"Are you allergic to penicillin?" I asked for the third time. Again no intelligible answer.

"No use," I said to the nurse. "Find someone who can speak Spanish."

The girl looked like a flower, a tropical flower. You couldn't say she was smiling, for that was the natural expression of her face, the face of a shiny bird or some other gentle, animated creature.

We found someone who claimed to know Spanish.

"Ask her whether she's allergic to penicillin. Make sure she understands you. It's very important."

The interpreter put the question to her in several (in fact, too many) sentences, and the girl answered in her broken English, "I not speak Spanish. . . . I Filipino."

Slowly we pieced together her story. Her boy friend had brought her to the clinic; he was on the men's side himself, with the same problem. And he spoke English. We sent a nurse over and got all the information we needed. He did have gonorrhea.

She let me take her blood without any difficulty, looking around her with big, shiny, slightly bewildered eyes. But to undress for the examination posed quite a problem: it turned out that she was having her period and had this morning put in a fresh Tampax. The American Tampax is of such a size that it can hardly be used by those small Pacific girls. How she had inserted it I do not know. But she was unable to get it out, especially standing on one foot in the middle of the room. Finally, with the help of two nurses, she succeeded.

Then she was put on the table. But when I approached her naked, spread-out legs, she jumped up, almost falling off the table. She could not understand our Western ways and suffered agonies over this exposure. Finally we subdued her, and she lay down like a small, sacrificial animal.

She turned out to be positive for gonorrhea. I tried to explain this to her as best I could and, before she got dressed, shot two injections of penicillin, one into each side of her miniature buttocks. She turned her heavy (*fauve*) head from one side to the other, murmuring in agony, "Oh, my God, oh, my God!" I thought she was going to collapse.

After that she vanished into the toilet.

Our toilets are a delicate subject. We do not want the patients, some perhaps on the verge of shock after needles and penicillin, to lock themselves in. A simple solution would be to take off the locks. But whose competence would that be? Perhaps the Commissioner's? And how would you reach the Commissioner? We have a handyman, but he isn't really a handyman, and he doesn't speak English, and as for the tools, no one knows where they are kept.

So it happened that the Filipino girl stepped into the toilet, locked herself in, and remained there for what seemed an eternity. (As it later turned out, she had been struggling to insert a fresh Tampax.) To all my knocks and shouts she made no answer, which was a logical defense on her part. I felt sure that she had collapsed and was about to break in the door (or break my shoulder) when she finally stepped out: pale, exhausted, with that eternal smile on her Oriental face.

59

Directly after the Filipino, two women came in together, both Chinese. One young, broad-faced, and sturdy; the other old, withered, used-up. The young woman was pregnant. Just arrived from Hong Kong and speaking no English, she was under the care of a Chinese doctor, who had sent her to us for the required blood test, under the protection of his old crone of a nurse.

As I was going through my routine, the young woman looked straight at me—a strong, untamed creature, subdued perhaps, but not overcome. She did not cry, she did not complain, she asked no questions. She did everything that I, through her chaperone, told her to do. I could make out no emotion, neither fear nor approval, in her attitude. I could not even tell whether she understood what I was trying to do. I had decided to take also a smear from her vagina (just in case, since she had so recently arrived from Hong Kong, where love is dangerous).

She spread her strong legs and let me do what was necessary. Her legs were tremendously muscular, and I had the impression that if she suddenly locked them on me, she could easily break my arms. All in all, I was confronted by an imperturbable, elementary force, seemingly controlled, yet not to be swayed or changed.

She was supposed to come back after a week for the results of the tests, but she did not appear. Three weeks later a particularly conscientious old nurse (she worked part-time, more for pleasure than from need, and could afford to be conscientious) came across her chart, which in heavily red-underlined notes stated that her test was highly positive for syphilis. The nurse immediately tried to get in touch with the Chinese doctor, whose card was attached to the chart. At the given address no such doctor had an office. "Don't worry, we'll find her," our chief investigator cheerfully proclaimed. "What do you mean, don't worry?" the conscientious nurse retorted. "This woman is in her seventh month. We must worry."

But that strong, wild creature had vanished in New York, exactly as if it were Hong Kong. Perhaps she had indeed returned there, together with the doctor.

60

Our clinics are plastered with posters. Madison Avenue, through different private agencies and pharmaceutical concerns, has been brought in to help us. Here are some samples:

YOU CAN'T HIDE FROM VENEREAL DISEASE
for information call 269-5300

V.D. STRIKES ONE PERSON EVERY TWO MINUTES

LA VERDAD SOBRE SÍFILIS Y GONORREA
(a pamphlet)

MOST IMPORTANT: DON'T CATCH SYPHILIS OR GONORRHEA
the best way to make sure you don't catch
those diseases is by clean living

DON'T PLAY AROUND WITH SEX

DON'T BE A TARGET FOR V.D.

HOW DO YOU KNOW YOU DON'T HAVE V.D.?

SPREAD THIS UGLY STORY AROUND

These and similar grimly humorous messages greet the wretched citizen who comes to our Health Centers.

The centers are fairly new buildings (in Queens I noted a date of construction: 1939). I am sure hundreds of thousands of dollars were spent searching for the most functional architectural design. But our toilets, as a rule, are filthy, often clogged and overflowing with gonorrheal urine. It is a miracle for a patient to find a working fountain if he wants a drink. The door handles are wet and dirty—polluted. As for the elevator, one never knows whether it is in, or out of, order.

In Harlem, where the clinic is on the sixth floor, the elevator moves so slowly that once inside you cannot tell which way it is going and whether it is moving at all. It stops on every floor, the door opens and closes with excruciating slowness, and if some dubious individual joins the rider and proceeds to mug him, no one could possibly come to his help.

We do have personnel to clean and wash and scrub the place at regular intervals. Yet the over-all impression is of dirt, chaos, and neglect. Apparently that's how things always turn out to be in New York City.

Of course, it would be asking too much to have piped-in Beethoven symphonies while the patients wait their turn. Some good souls did want to brighten the atmosphere and hung up huge photos of movie actors. Jackie Gleason, the Marx Brothers, Princess Grace of Monaco look down at us. Strangely enough, these decorations, too, add to the funereal atmosphere.

In most of our clinics women and men sit together in the same waiting room, all facing the VERDAD SOBRE SÍFILIS. You get used to anything! They sit on the benches like the dead in *Our Town*.

I don't know what could really change this atmosphere. Flowers? Paintings? Once in a while a fellow walks in with a guitar and, while he waits, begins to strum and sing. That does something to all of us. But this is spontaneous—not planned by the Central Office.

Once, I came into the waiting room and saw the nurses'

aides setting up a small new desk; they covered it with a paper cloth and set a small vase with artificial flowers in the center.

"They want some decoration," a sober, middle-aged black employee explained, "so here it is—decoration."

61

The man was clearly in a state of anxiety.

"What a sucker I am. . . . At sixty-five, can you believe it? Last Sunday she invited me for a drink, and we went to bed. After that it struck me: 'Gee, she let me enter her too easily; she must be one of those, you know.' The druggist gave me some ointment, and I squeezed it into my opening, and it's been burning like hell ever since."

"What is she, a whore?" I asked.

"No, a widow who probably needs some extra cash."

62

They sit there, for hours and hours. In the spring the sun shines outside, and every little group of trees seems a park. But they must wait inside the dismal mill. They are wet and itchy, disgusted and frightened. But the attraction between the sexes is great; no sooner are they cured than they start all over and then come back to us for new treatment. Despite all the tortures of the examination, the needles and the massive drugging, despite all their complaints, the impression is that most of them (especially the males) deep down somewhere feel that "it's worth it."

Of course, quite often they say the opposite. And they also think that it's inevitable, that "it has to happen." As one adolescent told me: "It's like paying taxes. If you want to live in New York, you pay high taxes and you are exposed to all kinds of violence and accidents."

However, the taxes are not evenly distributed. For some they are exorbitant. A youth sticks out his neck—or rather his penis—for the first time and right away gets syphilis. That really is cruel, or so it seems. But eventually, after going through a stage of fright and despair, they somehow accept it as a fact of life.

In the hall, at the information booth, a clerk distributes numbers to our clients. Thence, in one particular clinic, the women go to the right and the men to the left wing. Quite often one sees a young couple standing in the middle of the hall, both unkempt, with bushy manes and dirty-looking (to an outsider), frozen in an embrace, waiting for their numbers to be called. Did he give it to her? Did she give it to him? In a little while they will unfold their stories and, in the process, tell all kinds of lies. But here and now they keep their tight embrace, they forgive and ask for forgiveness, they make peace.

63

I usually work fast and efficiently. ("If you *have* to do it, do it quickly!" goes for doctors as well as for hangmen.) I plunge the big needle in without delay or preliminaries, since no speeches can make it smaller or softer. I am through very quickly, and the patient, after a painful grimace, sighs with relief. "Is that all?" they ask, and smile, satisfied. But some curse, complain, and threaten to write to the Central Office about my brutality.

I have noticed that if a patient is particularly dirty and smelly or ugly and dumb, I do my job somewhat sloppily. I do it as if I were holding my nose with one hand, which, spiritually, is indeed the case.

Here is a monstrosity: a female who has lost her human appearance, exposed to me in her most intimate and repulsive aspect. It smells bad—I wish I were far away, I wish she were far away. And she (it is usually a she, though it sometimes happens with a male, too), she feels it and "transfers" it. She complains to the Central Office of roughness, brutality, unprofessional behavior. She wants revenge for a metaphysical humiliation of which she is well aware. In short, she wants me, if not to admire her, at least to approve (physically).

64

What you see most during a two-and-a-half-hour session is genitals. Female and/or male. They are different and similar. Actually there exist only two sexual organs: one collective penis and one eternal vagina.

This penis, of course, may be smaller, bigger, more miserable or triumphant than another, but the differences among all of them are negligible, and their proprietors are far from proud when they expose them to me. In fact, at this moment the organ seems completely insignificant, and the owner, perhaps viewing it with detachment for the first time, is aware of this. Rotating his former pride and joy in front of my face, he looks at it with a sort of surprised contempt. (I am convinced that the so-called phallic cult is an invention, an erroneous interpretation.)

As for the female counterpart, it may be clean or garbage-like, it may stink or be perfumed, it may be dilated like that of a cow or virginally tiny, angry-red or gently pink—but here, too, there is only one collective vulva.

If one cuts a strawberry into halves, takes one half and splits the lower end, opening it up, one has the picture of what I face when placed between the spread legs of a female patient. (All, of course, subject to ethnological, social, and cultural factors.)

The one collective penis is, metaphysically, always stretched out toward its vulvar counterpart—sucked in by it, despite all outward personal, intellectual, and spiritual preferences. Such an overwhelming blind instinct fills me with pity. Love, it seems, has nothing to do with this drive.

Incidentally, to speak to my clients about love is very risky. It makes them laugh, as does the mention of duty, sin, or religion. They laugh, but all the same, some of them feel a sudden sympathy for me. They think I am a sucker. They even say so. But they come and shake hands with me in the end. And then my only hope is that by now the gonococci on their fingers have dried up.

65

The percentage of "no-speak-English" people is enormous in our V.D. establishments. Most of them, naturally, are Spanish-speaking. The lack of communication is very taxing on the doctor, who, before aggressive treatment, would like to get the patient's history. The stories they tell through our volunteer interpreters are always ambiguous and often dangerously so.

His wife came to the clinic the day before and was treated for syphilis. He does not know anything, he does not understand anything, he only smiles meekly, nods frequently, and, as far as the tests go, doesn't have the disease.

"What's your work? Your occupation?"

"Nothing. No work, no occupation," the interpreter explains, while the patient continues to nod and smile. I classify him S 90, which means epidemiological syphilis, and give him his first shot of penicillin (2,400,000 units).

Of course, before embarking on this, I had asked, "Are you allergic to penicillin?"

And he had answered first "Yes," then "No," and finally "I don't know." He could refuse the needle; he could refuse the tests. I don't believe it is constitutional to force American citizens to submit to treatments and injections. But simple people usually do submit. They think they have to.

66

This "no-speak-English" boy told me a long and incoherent story, which I interpreted as follows: a doctor had recently examined him and said that he was sick, very sick, and must run to a public-health clinic.

No complaints, no symptoms. After having taken his blood, I was about to get rid of him when a sharp investigator came up with the information that the boy was getting married the following week. The private doctor had made a test and found the result suspicious.

It also turned out that a good friend of the future bridegroom had, the day before, been treated at our clinic for syphilis. At this point the patient began to talk in English, not perfectly but quite adequately. In police stations, courtrooms, and other public agencies, islanders, for some reason, start out by playing dumb or even pretending to be completely illiterate.

Now this boy, too, wanted immediate treatment for syphilis. Despite his new-found eloquence I refused. Why did he have to get married next Tuesday? Why could he not wait for the results of the test?

Despite his polite nodding I felt that he hated me, just as he hated policemen, judges, priests, and storekeepers.

67

She is a heroin addict. An unprepossessing, pitifully pale, artificial blonde. No veins! And when, after almost an hour's hard work, I finally entered a tiny vein and began to draw blood, she very casually took off the tourniquet, messing up the entire procedure. "Look what you did to my arm," she moaned, showing me the puncture. My entire heroic effort was annihilated. I glared at her. She sat there, close to me, as if behind a wall, a glass wall.

Syphilis and addiction go hand in hand: when they are high, women really don't care about anything and throw themselves at the first chance; the same when they need money for a fix. And then there is, of course, the vicious circle that heroin addicts very often show a *false* positive reaction for syphilis. Quite a problem for us.

68

"You have syphilis," I told him.

He was a small, frail Puerto Rican, pale and undernourished. He took a deep breath, turned around, and dashed to the exit. After a little while he came back, bringing a girl with him: a tiny, emaciated, pretty Latin. As they approached, they exchanged some words and I heard her say, very womanly and tenderly, "You see, I told you."

What could she have possibly told him on their way here? That she has it? Or that he has it? But certainly that she loves him and wants him.

The boy put his arm around her shoulder, gently, protectively, and looked at me as if ready for execution.

"Both of you will be treated," I said. "We'll cure you. But first she, too, has to register."

Crossing the hall later, I noticed them several times while they were still waiting to register her. If for some reason we ever had to send a sample human couple to another planet, to show what such a couple looks like, what it expresses, to demonstrate its indivisibility, I wouldn't mind sending them: they'd do!

69

The boy, wild-haired, quite dirty, with an arrogant smile and a cigarette in his mouth, looked straight at me as if asking for a fight. The type of a Parisian *gavroche*—except that he was colored, probably Puerto Rican.

"I think I got a venereal disease," he announced without taking the cigarette out of his mouth.

"Why do you think so?"

"My friends told me about the girl. . . ."

"Do you have any symptoms? Any signs? Sores? Burning?"

"No, I have no symptoms." He dropped the word quite casually.

"How old are you?"

"Fourteen."

I could find nothing wrong with him, at least from the medical point of view.

"The results of the blood test won't be back for a week. In the meantime it would be a good idea to find out some more about this girl. She may have a file here. Perhaps we've treated her."

I called in an investigator, who very efficiently began by asking for the girl's name and address. The boy turned his back on him and asked me, "Do I have to tell?"

"It would help, but you don't have to."

"In that case, I'm not telling," retorted the little *gavroche* or musketeer from Harlem.

70

He plays the French horn. He is young and gifted and expects special treatment from me. But I am mad, really mad. Three weeks ago he came with a gonorrhea, which we cured. Now he is back, explaining, "I must have gone with the wrong girl. It started all over again."

"What are you, a dog? Can't you at least discriminate?"

He tries to stand up to me: "I'm not a dog. You can't talk to me that way. You have no right to call me that."

"That's just the point. You're not a dog, but you behave like one. And that I find disgusting."

While waiting for the result of the smear we start a neutral conversation. He used to play only classical music. Now he likes contemporary Americans. He's still good at Vivaldi. Do I like Tchaikovsky?

"No, I like Chopin. Actually, I like the piano most of all."

"Oh." He is surprised and somehow offended, for his horn.

"I like wind instruments, too," I say conciliatorily. "You see, air in Greek is *pneuma*, as in pneumatic. This word also stands for spirit, for spirituality. To be good, a horn player must be spiritually advanced."

He laughs—a young, energetic, healthy-looking black.

"How old are you?"

"Twenty-four."

The smear is positive. I give him a horse-size dose of penicillin.

"Look here . . ." I begin.

But he interrupts with a friendly smile: "I know, I know. Pneumatic!"

Later, crossing the waiting room, I noticed a very attractive young colored woman with a proud profile and tightly plaited hair engaged in a loud, intense conversation with my "pneumatic" customer. Eventually I called a number to which she responded.

"Having a good time here?" I asked.

"This I resent," she answered angrily. "This is very inconsiderate of you."

During the examination she told me that she was studying sociology and that she saw nothing wrong in behaving naturally in a health clinic. Whose business was it whether she had T.B. or V.D.? "There is no difference," she said.

"For some reason I feel that in a V.D. clinic the sexes should be separated, and if the waiting room is as stupidly arranged as here, women and men should sit apart and not socialize," I answered.

But she quoted some popular sociologist who seems to disagree with me. This spoiled, good-looking girl was also intelligent.

She had come in with a note from the physician in charge, prescribing a shot of penicillin. And yet her chart showed all tests negative.

"What's the story?" I asked.

The story was the usual one. Her boy friend had gone to a private doctor, who treated him for gonorrhea. He told her to go to the clinic.

"How strange," I said. "What kind of boy friends are those? He goes to a private doctor and sends you to the public clinic. It seems to me it should be the other way around."

"I myself chose the health clinic," said the sociologist. "The private doctor makes no tests. He just gives you a shot of penicillin and you pay."

"Well, perhaps you've a point there. But since your tests are negative, why should you get penicillin?"

"Because he is sick. And I had contact with him," she explained. "I have a child and want to protect her."

"But you can't be sure about your boy friend. As you say, the doctor didn't make any tests. Why not wait till next week, when we'll have the result of your culture? Then everything will be clear. Meanwhile you must behave yourself, you understand."

She accepted my point of view (the chief had probably told her the same thing before) and was about to leave when she wheeled around and asked, "By the way, can I have intercourse with my husband?"

The sudden appearance of a husband in the picture threw me off balance for a moment. Apparently I'm not up on modern sociology.

"No, you cannot have intercourse with your husband," I answered, looking with fear at her beautiful, intelligent, capricious face.

"Not even if he puts on a condom?"

"Not if he puts on a dozen. Abstinence at this stage is as important as antibiotics."

"Yes, they say so; no sex, no spices, no liquor."

"That's correct. Except that 'no sex' also includes no sexual stimulation, no excitement, no erection. That's what it means."

She looked at me, slightly puzzled. Sex, she had thought, meant only copulation.

"Take good care of your child," I said, rather unconvinced. Frankly, I didn't see how she could.

72

"May I close the door?" he asked, stepping into my small room.

"Of course, by all means," I answered unenthusiastically. The room is tiny, there is no air conditioning, and the way I see it, the patients have no real secrets to confide to me. A moment ago they all huddled together, but once inside even the most exhibitionist of them wants privacy.

After we had ascertained that he had a recent syphilitic ulcer and would need thorough treatment, he said to me, "I'm a writer. It may all be for the best. One needs such dramatic experiences."

"Of course, of course," I agreed cautiously. I did not trust his square head and the transparent colorlessness of his eyes. And there was something strange in his slow, dignified movements.

"What do you write about?" I asked.

"About great things. Unorthodox things. Not pleasant for the average man." He laughed with a bitter and triumphant air. "Here is a piece I just started while waiting for my Dark Field. Of course it needs polishing." And he handed me a page, one paragraph of which I copied while he was being interviewed by an investigator.

"Never again will we do such intricate revision of the subsequent aversion in the dormitory which has not yet found the needed expression of prediluminary substance since forever fighting in the mud of subhuman existence one must try to subdue instincts worse than the death of death. . . ."

"Is there a way of sending this fellow to a psychiatrist?" I inquired of our chief. He only looked at me disgustedly, as so often. During the vacation months we are really very busy.

73

"Two weeks ago I got a shot of penicillin, in prison, at Rikers Island. And now I've started to drip again." He was a twenty-two-year-old black, with shining eyes, alive and open to communication. His arms were all in "tracks."

"Are you a junkie?" I asked.

"I used to be. But now I'm off the hook."

"What do you think of methadone?"

"I'm trying to join a program. It's not easy to get in."

"Do you think it's good?"

"I want to try."

I did not ask him why he had been locked up; his was probably a routine crime. "How do they treat you there, in prison?" I inquired.

He thought for a moment and then, slowly, deliberately, said, "If you behave, if you behave yourself," he said, a meaningful glance in his shining eyes, "they treat you all right." And he nodded.

I could easily figure out that if you did not "behave yourself" they treated you very badly. I gave him his shot. That was all I could do for him.

74

His Dark Field was positive. He was still sitting on the table, protecting his scratched, oozing penis with his arms.

"You have syphilis," I said.

He looked at me with an absent, blank look, which, on the one hand, proved that he could not grasp the meaning of my words completely and, on the other hand, that he suddenly realized something was wrong, altogether wrong, in his past. How often have I seen this agonized look and wished I could help. Encourage them to start anew, to live better. But I always know, despite my pity, how little there is in my power to do.

"Is it a serious case?" he asked. (Many ask this question.)

"It's a typical case," I answered. "We'll treat you, and if you follow our instructions you'll be cured." (I don't want them to feel too secure. . . .) "I understand your wife is here, too," I continued.

"She's not my wife." His eyes, although full of painful hatred, were those of a tortured lamb. "She's only my common-law wife, and she gave it to me."

"We'll treat her, too," I promised.

But that did not seem to comfort him.

75

Simultaneously we got two positive Dark Fields—husband and wife.

"Who gave it to whom?" I asked the doctor who was taking care of the couple.

"Oh, I never ask any questions," he answered with surprise. "It's not good for the physician to get involved."

76

He was like a full-grown baboon: strong, red-cheeked, with no eyebrows. I wouldn't say that he was perfectly adjusted to survival. No, the main impression was that he was, primarily, adjusted to getting all kinds of pleasure, and only pleasure, out of life. He had come, summoned by a letter from our clinic; one of our newly treated syphilitics had named him as a contact.

"Are you allergic to penicillin?"

"I don't know," he said belligerently.

"Have you ever had V.D.?"

"I don't believe so."

"Have you any complaints now, any symptoms?"

"How should I know?"

There are such "strong" characters, entire ethnic groups,

menially employed or exploited minorities, which, owing to their historical experience, find it best to play it dumb and never to give a straight answer.

But this one surely overdid it.

When I asked him, "Was this contact a woman or a man?" he answered slowly, as if making a genuine effort to recall, "I really don't remember."

77

"If I got it again I'll kill him," she said, her small, childish face, despite her bitterness and tears, still somehow smiling. On her chart was a stamp: MINOR. And indeed, she was only sixteen years old. Two and a half years ago we had treated her for syphilis. Now she had come because her boy friend, who recently "got his shots" at our clinic (it was not clear whether for syphilis or gonorrhea), had told her to have a checkup, too.

"I know the girl who gave it to him," she informed me, obviously getting great satisfaction out of the fact that she was not dumb.

"What's the name of your boy friend?" I asked. My idea was to find his chart and thus to solve several problems at once.

"I don't know," she said, laughing, "I always call him Tony."

78

On a long weekend she went to visit her boy friend in Atlanta; now he had called to tell her that he was under treatment and that she had better have a checkup for clap right away.

"How is Atlanta in the spring?"

"Oh, beautiful."

"Did you ever have a venereal disease?"

"No, never."

"How old are you?"

"Twenty-eight. Oh, that hurts. Can't you be a little gentler? The private doctors are so gentle."

"How do you know?"

"I used to go for vaccination when I was a child."

"And you didn't cry then?"

"Oh, yes, I did, but it was so nice."

79

All three of them arrived together: a man, a woman, and a child of about four. A common-law family of six years' standing. Recently the couple decided to get married. They took the routine blood test at a private office, and his blood showed up weakly reactive for syphilis.

"Yes," he confirmed, "eleven years ago I got bad blood in this country and was treated."

"How about me, am I sick, too? And what about my child?" she kept asking.

We took new blood tests.

"If your blood shows a disease we'll treat you," I told her. "Don't worry."

"And the boy?"

"If your blood is bad we'll test his blood, too, but only then. Don't worry, we'll take care of all of you."

"I want to get married and immediately divorce him so that he has to pay for the child," she explained with cold rage, in his presence.

What an irony: an ideal couple with a nice child. After six years of life together they decide to legalize their union.

And it's just because of this reasonable step that their relationship falls apart.

80

"Es alérgica Usted a la penicilina?" That's what I am supposed to ask when I need this vital information. But I guess for a simple Puerto Rican there is no difference between "allergic" and *"alérgica"*—he understands neither word. First he says "Yes," then he says "No," and finally, "I don't know," all this smiling happily.

Simple people often take the word "allergic" to mean whether they like to take it, whether they accept it. "Are you allergic to penicillin?" I ask. *"Es Usted alérgica a la penicilina?"* And they answer enthusiastically, "Yes, yes."

It doesn't mean a thing.

81

These two women were Canadian. French-speaking.

I would never have believed that there are Canadians who do not speak a word of English. Yet one of them, the younger and more attractive one, apparently did not. The other, heavily painted and decrepit, spoke English as well as French. (In fact, both spoke a decent French, not the Canadian kind, where a car is called a *char*.)

They wanted to check up on syphilis.

"Why?"

"My sister went with such a man, and I sleep in the same bed with her. Besides, I, too, had relations with him, before," the older woman explained. She looked like a whore—a conventional, old-fashioned whore.

More I could not find out. It looked to me as if the younger woman, freshly arrived from Montreal, had been put into business by her "sister." Whatever it was, they seemed figures sprung from the pages of a short story by Maupassant.

I could not find anything wrong with them and, reluctantly, let them loose.

A week later the tests showed that both had active syphilis.

82

"Sit down and roll up your right sleeve," said the nurse.

"Can I speak to the doctor first?" the man asked. He was still young but with a tendency toward early middle age: balding, already with a slight paunch.

"Yes, what is it?" I anticipated the nurse before she had a chance to have things "her way." Our nurses have all been "in the system" for years and years and do not easily brook interference in their routine.

"You see, Doctor . . ." and then followed his story.

Monday night he went with a woman to her apartment. Soon he got "disgusted," but she insisted, and he was obliged to make love in an unnatural way—"You know, in her mouth," he whispered. After that, even more disgusted, he left. Now he is about to go back to Rochester, where he has a wonderful family, and naturally he wants to make sure that he did not pick up a bad disease.

"We'll get the results only in one week," I said.

"Oh." He became quite agitated. "I can't allow you to write to my home. Tell me, what are the chances I picked up something from her?"

"Frankly—nil," I said. "But since you worry so much about your family you really shouldn't get involved in such situations."

"I see what you mean, Doctor. Thank you very much." And with a hearty laugh he walked out. I bet that on his next business trip he won't miss a similar "disgusting" opportunity.

83

The young man of twenty-four, heavy-set, pleasant-looking, with a Spanish name but obviously born in New York, refused to have a blood test.

"I had it a month ago; that's enough."

"Then why are you here?" I asked.

"I have some trouble," he said.

"Since when?"

"For two years."

It evolved that he was about to get married and wanted some help before. "You know what I mean!"

I didn't, and he was obliged to enlighten me.

"I can't get a decent erection, Doctor. How long will it take you to straighten me out?"

He really believed in science.

84

A heavy, muscular fellow, who could be a truck driver or construction worker, except for his clean, smooth hands.

"You are really good at it," he said, when I was drawing the 5 c.c. of blood.

"I'm sure you're as good in your own field," I said, to repay the compliment.

"I only wish I were."

"What's your profession?"

"I'm a salesman." He mentioned the brand name of some household articles. "Before I know it I get involved in sex with the housewives, and there go my time and money."

Poor housewives. There they sit all day, waiting for the bell to ring. They're waiting for an ideal salesman and for all he has to offer. . . .

"I feel like killing her," he said thoughtfully.

"After all, she got it from you, didn't she?" I countered.

"From me?" He was indignant.

"All right. From some other fellow. What's the difference? It's a vicious circle. Do you understand: a vicious circle."

"Yes, I know what you mean," he said, unconvinced. "When should I come back?"

"A week from today."

"A week from today is Good Friday!" the nurse said.

85

This morning the Health Officer, who is the chief of the Center, summoned all doctors for a briefing.

1. We must sign arrivals and departures *separately* and give exact time (to the minute) of both. We will be paid according to these entries.

2. There have been many complaints to the Central Office. The patients claim they are being treated like garbage. The Commissioner and his deputies hate such complaints. We must be polite with the patients. There is no excuse for not being polite. It appears that some patients were told that if they are able to fuck, they must be able to stand a needle. This the Central Office does not like at all.

During the ensuing discussion we (the doctors) brought up the point that the patients are very annoyed by the amount of time they waste waiting around in the clinic. Instead of calling the patient and processing him in one or two stages, the routine, established years ago, calls for twelve separate steps. The paper work is much too heavy, which, considering the background of our clerks, creates an absurd situation.

61

"That can't be helped," the Officer said curtly.

"If only the Commissioner or a deputy could once come and see for himself. What would you say of a general who never visits his advance battalions, the ones in action?" I ventured.

But he cut me short. "Gentlemen, it's getting late. I must warn you that, besides myself, some of the nurses and investigators are also watching your arrivals and departures. We are in for austerity. They are trying to save every buck they can. So watch out!"

86

People come to us from all over the world to learn how V.D. control is organized in New York City. Thus, the Health Department advised us that in the middle of March a doctor from New Zealand was expected and should be shown all our facilities and procedures. "We trust that the arrangement will provide a meaningful and fruitful experience for the visitor," the letter concluded.

It was with fear and trembling that I watched the brass conducting the New Zealander through our premises. The best pages of Kafka, Beckett, and Ionesco hardly equal the absurdity of N.Y.C. arrangements. Facing is the official scheme of PRESENT PATIENT FLOW to which we are obliged to adhere.

From this scheme, which might have been worked out by the Scholastics of the Middle Ages, the reader can easily see that out of the twelve or thirteen steps through which the poor V.D. customer is forced to move, one half of the total (steps 2, 4, 6, 8, 10, and 12) require him to go back to the waiting room, sit down, and wait again. This *danse macabre* adds at least one hour to the patient's waiting time, besides being absurd and humiliating. If we processed him in two or three steps, our work would be more efficient and humane.

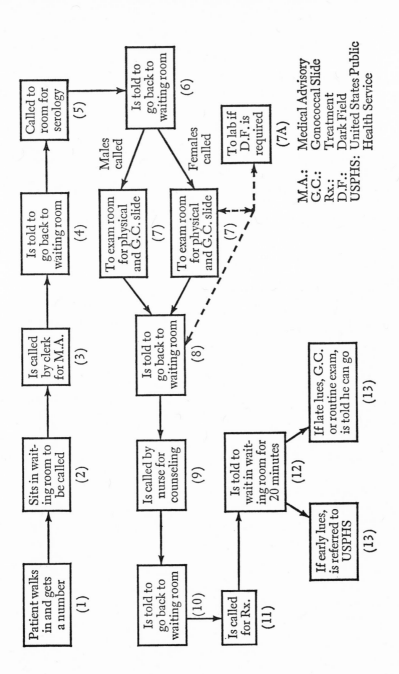

Patient walks in and gets a number (1)

Sits in waiting room to be called (2)

Is called by clerk for M.A. (3)

Is told to go back to waiting room (4)

Called to room for serology (5)

Is told to go back to waiting room (6)

Males called

Females called

To exam room for physical and G.C. slide (7)

To exam room for physical and G.C. slide (7)

To lab if D.F. is required (7A)

Is told to go back to waiting room (8)

Is called by nurse for counseling (9)

Is told to go back to waiting room (10)

Is called for Rx. (11)

Is told to wait in waiting room for 20 minutes (12)

If late lues, G.C. or routine exam, is told he can go (13)

If early lues, is referred to USPHS (13)

M.A.: Medical Advisory
G.C.: Gonococcal Slide
Rx.: Treatment
D.F.: Dark Field
USPHS: United States Public Health Service

I once had the temerity to propose that the patients be treated directly after examination and lab test, *i.e.*, to initiate step 11 directly after step 7. The reaction was as if I had suggested a Russian revolution. All the ignorant and unqualified personnel (and they are in the majority) considered their positions in jeopardy, since routine is their only trusted ally.

The official explanation why the patient has to wait for treatment until he is "admitted" and his card written out is that if he were treated immediately he would walk out without waiting for his "admission card" and indoctrination (counseling). In most of the cases this does not apply: our patients like to be treated; they come again and again, ask many questions, and very often continue patiently waiting for hours, because nobody has told them that now they may leave.

After having been "admitted" and treated, the patient has to wait another twenty minutes in case he has any untoward reaction to the penicillin.

If, furthermore, one keeps in mind that our clerks take about fifteen to twenty minutes to admit a patient, and that when they have finally written out his papers, they do not rush to bring them to the doctor but accumulate three or four charts at a time, since, as they put it, "they are not messengers," then the absurdity of the patient-flow arrangement becomes obvious. Sometimes there are several doctors standing around, waiting for a chart to be filled out in order to do some work. The shortage is less of doctors than of intelligent, literate clerks.

I hope the doctor from New Zealand fully appreciated the merits of our organization. (She looked quite intelligent.)

87

Some time ago we received a letter from the Central Office, informing us that a certain Mr. N. "has been assigned by the Health Service Administration to review and make recommendations with regard to the activities of the Bureau of Venereal Disease Control. In connection with his assignment he will, during the next several months, be visiting, inspecting, and reviewing all of the Social Hygiene clinics.

"I am certain," continued the executive from the Central Office, "that all personnel will co-operate fully to facilitate Mr. N.'s analysis. I would strongly recommend that you take advantage of his visits to bring to his attention any and all suggestions that may facilitate our getting better service to patients and also to improve the working situation and morale of all health workers."

Would it not seem logical to ask those who are working there day in and day out for suggestions, analyses, and recommendations? Why hire a college graduate, even one with a master's degree (as this particular young man turned out to be), and pay him a substantial yearly salary for doing an absurd and futile job? What can he possibly see, understand, and improve by coming once or twice to the front lines, where we are fighting our day-by-day battles?

"Now you'll tell him the truth," I said to the physician in charge.

"What truth? What are you talking about?" that mild *Homo burocraticus* replied.

"That we need literate clerks, that the nurses and investigators are not doing their job, that the patients should be treated immediately after diagnosis, and not have to dance that eternal quadrille . . ."

"In any case, don't you talk to him," he told me. "I'm thirty-five years in the system. Leave it to me. He'll come, he'll look, he'll go. I've seen such wise guys, don't worry."

And indeed, when the tall young man with the good Harvard accent appeared and politely began to talk to all the supervisors, I realized that the last thing he wanted was a straight-from-the-shoulder story, and that it would be absolutely futile to tell him our grievances.

Incidentally, I never saw this six-footer again.

65

88

"Don't ever leave them alone in your room," the physician in charge said. "They'll steal anything."

So far I've caught only two patients of mine stealing. One had grabbed a bunch of used plastic disposable syringes, their needles bent and full of infectious material, which I had thrown into the trash can. The other was pocketing a couple of boxes of tetracycline.

When I refuse to give them the pills (because there is no direct indication), they think I'm cruel, stingy, stupid. I've sold out to the establishment, they say!

It is amazing how little people know about the possible harm and side effects of a wonder drug.

89

A boy of nineteen, slim, clean, intelligent, with curly hair and a mischievous smile. The adolescent Pushkin might have looked this way.

He was carrying a stack of textbooks under his arm. And we had three different charts for him; he had already had several bouts of gonorrhea, had been cured every time, and now he was back again.

I picked up two of his books: *Le Grand Meaulnes*, by Alain Fournier, and *Miracles*, by C. S. Lewis.

"As for books, you are on the right track," I said. He smiled.

He was studying history and sociology at Fordham. His French was quite good, and he intended to go to Europe the following year. A black, he was apparently from a good family—and that helped. (It always does.)

"Tell me, is it one girl who keeps giving you gonorrhea, or are there several?" He laughed but did not reply. "You see, if it's one girl and you care about her, you should bring her here and we'll treat her, too," I continued. Again he only laughed noncommittally. But about *Le Grand Meaulnes* he spoke freely, making it clear that he was familiar with all kinds of quests. He was a romantic, a dreamer, he said.

Since I did not want him to be a monthly repeater, I tried to impress on him that from too many shots he might develop an allergy to penicillin and that, someday, when he needed it badly, he wouldn't be able to take it.

This hit home. "How strange," he said, no longer smiling. "I never thought of that."

90

This was a contact syphilis: another patient had given his name as one of his (or her) recent companions.

"I have no symptoms whatsoever," he volunteered, apparently very much at ease, "and I have no idea who this person could be."

"Was it a man or a woman?" I asked. (This always gives an indication of where to look for a sore.)

"I don't know," he said. "It could be anything."

"What are you studying?" It was obvious that he was a student.

"Philosophy."

"I never could understand bisexuals," I said. "To a homosexual the experience with a woman must seem a nightmare, just as to a heterosexual a man in bed is repulsive. How do you manage to derive pleasure from both situations?"

"All such definitions and abstractions and generalizations have nothing to do with the individual case," he said very casually.

"Yes, I'm asking about your personal experience, which, I assume, is common to other bisexuals, too."

He looked at me with approval, small and agile, red-bearded, about twenty-seven years old. "I am always taken in by the person," he said, "by the personality. If it happens to be a woman, okay for the woman. If it's a man, I'm charmed by the man."

"And no preference?" I asked, not convinced.

"No preference," he answered, avoiding my eyes.

"Who is your favorite philosopher?"

"Marcuse."

"And how is Socrates doing on the campus these days?"

"He's all right; he'll survive a couple more semesters. Say, Doc"—here he became serious—"I just got shots for typhus and cholera. Would your penicillin interfere with it?"

"It might. Why did you have those shots? Are you going to Asia?"

"No, I just came back from East Africa."

"Abyssinia?"

"No, Tanganyika."

"Oh, they are very radical there, aren't they?"

"Not very." He dismissed them.

Later, walking through the hall, I heard a middle-aged, poorly dressed Negro woman say, "And how about Romeo and Juliet?" And a soft masculine voice answering something. I looked around; yes, it was the bisexual red-bearded philosopher, having an intellectual conversation about the Shakespeare Festival with this poorly dressed older woman.

But why Romeo and Juliet? And what about *Le Grand Meaulnes*? Simple coincidence? How many questers and dreamers are there among our patients?

91

He looked like a hermaphrodite on an ancient Greek amphora: tall and strong, but ageless and of no definite sex.

"How old are you?" This always seems to be a good opening.

"How old do you think I am?" he rather listlessly asked back.

"Forty-two?"

"Thank you." He smiled a bitter smile. "I'm forty-seven."

He was about to leave the room when the nurse picked up a heavy portfolio, which he had put on a chair.

"Is this your work?" she asked. "May I look?"

"Yes, you may."

She opened the portfolio and immediately began to compliment him. It was a collection of photographs: pictures of his sculptures and collages. As I understood it, he assembled different objects into abstract sculptures and collages, took pictures of these works, and exhibited (or sold) only the photographs. Indeed, the pictures did look good. (Exactly like other pictures of similar objects.)

"Do you like Moore?" I asked.

"Henry Moore," he corrected me, to make sure of his superiority. "Yes," he said with great deliberation, "I like him."

At the door he turned around and said to the nurse, "Thank you, you made this experience a little less painful."

Apparently there was nothing he could thank me for.

92

A homosexual whose blood test, after treatment for syphilis, was negative wanted to know whether it was 100 per cent sure that he was cured. I could not oblige him. I don't know. For all practical purposes we consider him cured. In twenty-five years from now there may be a more sensitive test that will disclose traces of the disease.

I told him so, and he got very angry. He wanted a clear-cut answer: yes or no. They all want a clear-cut answer. The homosexuals, the heterosexuals, and also the bisexuals.

93

He entered, swaying slightly and looking around him with shrewd caution. When he began to speak, it was as if he were putting on a stutter, a kind of defensive slowing down of speech, to give himself time to digest my questions. He was a Negro of about forty, with childish eyes and a meek, slightly sarcastic, understanding smile. He smelled of liquor.

"It's barely ten o'clock in the morning and you are already drunk," I said.

"When you live on the Bowery you wake up and start a pint of wine; otherwise you can't live on the Bowery."

"Why?" I asked sheepishly.

"You can't face it," he said, stuttering again.

"What do you do for a living?"

"Odd jobs. Mostly nothing," he explained, looking at me out of his serene, childish eyes.

In 1960 he was treated for syphilis on a state farm (a penal institution). But now he has come because he "drips."

"Do you like reading books?"

"Yes, I like to read. Why do you ask?" He seemed surprised.

"The way you express yourself, the words you use—and besides, since you have so much leisure time, reading would seem in order. There are fantastically good books, you know."

"Yes, I know."

"What have you read?"

"I've read Spinoza. And Shomshomshom . . ." he tried some German name, which might have been Schopenhauer. "I also read Freud."

"I know some very nice people near the Bowery, at the

Catholic Worker," I said. "Have you heard the name of Dorothy Day? They have a soup line, a reading room, and they publish a paper."

"Oh, yes, I know about Dorothy Day," he said, with a shrewd spark in his eyes. "Some people say that she is a mystical personality."

"She is my friend," I said proudly.

"I once went with my church to their farm on Staten Island and saw her. It was good. She is so calm." He looked up to the ceiling and his voice tried to convey a sensation of peace and quiet. "She never gets angry or sad."

"Why don't you go to their place on First Street?"

"I went a couple of times," he said, "but there are only kids around. They handle the soup line. When you ask for Dorothy they say, 'Dorothy is upstairs, sleeping.'" He laughed. "She cannot always be upstairs, asleep. Those kids are simply making fun of us."

"I once brought four gallons of California wine to their soup line on Easter Sunday and poured a cup for every guest," I told him.

"That's great," he answered, smiling his shrewd smile.

"What would you say the people there thought of me?" I asked, because for a long time I had been wanting to know.

"Well, it's always good to have a glass of wine, but they probably didn't think about you at all."

"Could they have thought that I'm a sucker?"

"Why?" He seemed surprised. But then he said, "Yes, they probably did think so. But what difference does it make?"

"You have clap," I told him. "We'll give you penicillin."

He magnanimously consented.

"Do you go often with women?" I asked.

"No, not often. When I have an extra dollar I get a woman; otherwise I don't bother."

"Have you always lived like that?"

"No, I was married. My wife died from diabetes."

"So it's after she died that you began to drink?" I was almost relieved to find an explanation for this waste of life.

"No. As a matter of fact, I drank much more when she was alive, and I drank hard liquor. I would come home from work and find her in a coma. That worried me. Now I drink only wine, and I can handle any amount."

He let down his pants, exposed his meager buttocks for the shots, and, smiling the same shrewd, childish smile, walked out—without any grudge against me, the establishment, or God Almighty.

94

He was a stocky little man, the kind that looks mature, even middle-aged, before thirty. He understood and spoke English, but took a long time to produce his answers. He was very cautious—probably life had taught him to be so.

"No, I never had syphilis, to the best of my knowledge."

Why, then, is his blood positive? He doesn't know.

"Have you ever had penicillin shots?"

"It's possible; I'm not sure."

"How many shots?"

No answer.

"Three or four or five?"

"Four or five."

"When was that?"

"Oh, about ten years ago."

"Could it be that you had syphilis at that time? Bad blood?"

The doctor from his Local had sent him to us because he showed a weak positive serological reaction. That could mean that he had syphilis, or that he had an immunological scar after having been treated for it, or that he had at some time or other contracted one of the tropical diseases that produce a false positive reaction. Or he might have been a drug addict.

There is a more sensitive serological test: the Fluorescent Treponemal Antibody test, FTA for short. For this, one has to send the sample to a special laboratory, and the result takes three weeks to come back. But what should I do with this little man meanwhile? Let him go home without treatment? I hate the idea of letting such obscure little males loose onto the streets of our city. I see Times Square seething with pale *Spirochaetae*, incessantly copulating, dividing, and reproducing. Give him the full treatment before being sure that he is dangerous?

Come to think of it, why pick exclusively on syphilis? What about dangerous ideas, ideological bombs, spiritual mines, intellectual traps? What about pornography? Forcible preventive medicine is *censorship!* Why accept this kind of censorship and fight the others?

95

As a general rule they blame someone for "giving it" to them. He blames her, she blames him. The female often begs me, "Tell him I don't have it, otherwise he won't believe me." In many cases there is a third party involved; the man (it mostly is the man) will call up and say to his girl, "You'd better go see a doctor. I'm sure I've got it." And the woman tells me, "I know who gave it to him."

It seems that no one can be blamed personally, individually. Often three or four or five persons are involved, and it becomes a circle, a vicious circle, of course. Nowhere is the *perpetuum mobile* of evil so evident as here. "Who gave it to whom?" is like the eternal question about the chicken and the egg.

This vicious circle can be broken only by an absolute stop, a radical abstention (besides penicillin), a six-week moratorium for everyone involved. How clear seem to me the scientific and beneficial implications of Lent! And yet a doctor is reluctant to speak about abstention. It sounds *moralistic*.

He arrived minutes before we closed the reception line. He came in with his bicycle: a nice, brand-new racing machine; English, I believe. He wheeled it into the hall, then into the waiting room, and finally, when I called his number, he pushed it into my narrow office, letting the back wheel stick out into the corridor and pulling the door half-shut.

Dry, neat, intent only on his own affairs, he gave his reasons for coming: the usual reasons of a neurotic. He didn't think he could possibly have V.D., but he wanted to make absolutely sure.

While I was busying myself over him taking the smear, he looked back and around to make sure that the front wheel of his bicycle hadn't vanished. After that, militaristically belted, a pack on his shoulders, he slowly, majestically, proceeded out with his shiny, whirring machine, through the waiting room to the hall, and into lower Manhattan; watched by all of us—doctors, patients, and nurses—with admiration and a kind of horror.

Several months later he came again. I recognized him immediately, because he carried a shiny bicycle wheel under his arm.

"What happened?" I asked, more concerned about the bicycle than about him. "Did your bicycle break down?"

"Oh, no. I take the front wheel off. That way anyone who wants to steal it can't just ride away; he'd have to carry it," he explained with equanimity.

This time he had to get the full treatment for gonorrhea.

97

She is sixteen. A high-school student. She thinks she contracted V.D. at Christmas but had no opportunity to check on it. Now, on her Easter vacation, she came to us.

"What kind of V.D. do you have in mind?"

"I don't know. Isn't it all the same?"

"No. There's syphilis, and there's gonorrhea. One is more serious than the other."

"I didn't know that," she said apologetically. She was a small, thin Italian girl, a good kid, with brilliant (probably hyperthyroidian) eyes.

Later she stopped me in the waiting room. Now she was relaxed and sure of herself (the test had been negative), and she said, "Could I perhaps get a job here for the summer? Even part-time would be all right. I like the atmosphere."

The nurses and clerks, who heard her, smiled, apparently flattered. They directed the girl to the Personnel Office on the clean, quiet, spacious third floor. I never saw her again.

98

It was the woman's second visit, and this time she brought her four-year-old daughter along. I had to check whether the mother was cured and make sure that the child had not contracted her gonorrhea. In certain parts of the city, particularly in Harlem, it is routine practice in such cases to take the little girls' smears, too.

The mother, it turned out, was still positive. The child was negative but very poorly kept. We decided to give the girl a preventive shot of penicillin, to play it safe. She put up quite a fight, flailing her arms and legs, crying and hitting out at the three of us. Just when I was plunging in the needle the mother asked whether I was sure that the girl needed this injection.

"No, I'm not sure at all," I answered, ready to curse.

We are expected to know everything, to be immaculate, to perform miracles. If only they realized how limited we are in our science, just trying to do our best, the best from the point of view of the present state of knowledge, and contributing quite a bit of harm along the way.

"How come I'm not cured yet?" the mother challenged me, ready to question my competence, if not that of the entire medical establishment.

She was a pale, intellectual-looking Negro woman, slim and quite attractive. A teacher, separated from her husband, she was taking courses at Fordham in order to qualify for high-school teaching.

"Well, your boy friend must be very tenacious." I tried to brush off her question with a joke.

"You're not kidding," she answered, smiling happily.

99

"He claims I gave it to him."

"And you claim he gave it to you?" I said.

"No, I really don't know."

"How important is it who gave it to whom?" I pursued, always eager to learn something.

"If you care about the fellow, it really doesn't matter," she answered after a moment's thought.

100

What a horror: these girls of twenty, attractive, slightly dirty, and unemployed.

"I'm not working right now" is their answer. Some of them are studying art, or so they say; some are models or dancers with no contract "right now."

They are very conscious of their genitals, and at the slightest "pimple" there, they come for a checkup. It is striking how well they know the situation of the sore and the moment when it first appeared. They have a peculiar way of smiling shyly when they spread their legs.

101

Hardly inside the clinic, the young white woman collapsed. We put her on a table and called the police and an ambulance. The police brought her Negro boy friend along, from whom we got the information that she had taken pills.

"How many pills did you take?" the officer asked her very gently, over and over.

"What kind of pills?" I inquired. The boy friend and the policeman simultaneously said something that sounded like "Dance." It took me a while to realize that they meant "downs," the opposite of up pills, or pep pills. "Downs" usually are phenobarbital, Nembutal, Seconal.

The Negro friend, a thin six-footer with an intelligent face, obviously embarrassed by the attention of doctors and police, nevertheless held her hand and kept whispering, "Alice, you're all right, aren't you, Alice?"

And Alice, pale as a woman who has just given birth, looked at him expressionlessly and without an answer.

Since her pulse was good and we were all anxious to get rid of her as quickly as possible, I let the officer take her in his car without waiting for the ambulance.

102

A methadone center opened at one of our clinics. Months ago I had applied for a job with them. It seemed to me that since I work in the same place and since a good fifth of our patients are junkies, I would be particularly suited for such a job. Also, it happens they pay two or three times as much as Social Hygiene. But that's exactly why I didn't get the job!

In preparation for the opening the whole clinic was freshly painted and the V.D. division pushed into a far corner. The methadone clinic was painted all in yellow, our part in two colors: half purple, half pink. Apparently purple for gonorrhea and pink for syphilis (or vice versa?).

103

Many patients have become used—at private offices or at clinics with poor technicians—to getting their needle right in the middle of the buttock. I give it in the upper lateral corner, as prescribed. Suspicious of any deviation from the routine and distrustful as they are of the establishment, they resent this: it hurts more and for a longer time, they claim. Often I am too rushed to explain to them that in the center, where they want it, the huge sciatic nerve runs down, and that one must not stick the needle in its vicinity.

So I stick my needle where I choose, and they are sure that I enjoy torturing them. They call me "Bruto," "Butcher," or, preferably, "Fucking bastard."

104

A woman's voice on the phone asked for one of my colleagues.

"I'm sorry, he's busy in another room," I answered. "Any message?"

"Don't give me that, go and fetch him," the bitchy voice called over the wire. I hung up, but the phone kept ringing.

When I told the supervisor of nurses about this call, she laughed. "Yes, I know, he has his problems, too."

"Was it his wife?" I wanted to know.

"I don't know, I doubt it," she said.

The emergence of this doctor, a man in his late fifties, in the role of persecuted and spied-on lover added a new dimension to our V.D. clinic.

105

Today is my birthday. Of course I haven't mentioned it to anyone around.

A rather arrogant young man comes in.

"Ah, that's the one who collapses," says the nurse. "You have to put him on the table before you give him the shot."

"Yes, yes," the youth affirmed with a smile. "I'm the one who collapses."

That smile of his, his superior air, and the pride he took in collapsing rubbed me the wrong way.

"If you fuck women you must be able to take a needle," I said.

"That's an offensive remark," he answered promptly. "And besides, I don't fuck women, I fuck men."

"That makes no difference. Anyway, you get your needle

like everybody else." I really hated his guts. "At your age I had been in two wars and I wasn't afraid of bullets." (As if that could prove anything.)

"Congratulations," he retorted with a "knowing" smile. "And how many people did you kill?"

"No more than you."

"Oh, leave me alone." He turned away, as if what I had said he had heard a thousand times and it was below his dignity to argue. "What kind of professional ethics is this, anyhow!"

"And what is your profession?" I asked quietly, preparing the syringe. "If it's no indiscretion."

"It *is* an indiscretion," he answered.

"I thought so," I said.

The needle is of steel or some other metal, and, regardless of your emotions and whether you like or detest the flesh into which you have to plunge it, it causes pain.

106

His veins were sclerosed. I shook my head in disapproval. The junkie understood and only smiled meekly.

I got the vein all right. As usual I asked, "What do you think of the Methadone Program?"

"It's good," he answered, without much conviction, "but I want to kick it straight."

He was a small, manly-looking fellow, about eighteen years old, probably Spanish. When it came to taking his smear he explained that it had to be an anal one. "Not from the front."

"So you have to straighten out twice," I said rather dejectedly. "I wish I could help you."

Again he smiled meekly and did not answer.

107

A fair, almost transparent adolescent with a positive Dark Field.

"I wanted to ask you . . ." he began. I knew what he wanted: assurance that after his shots of penicillin he would be completely cured.

"Yes," I said, "you'll be all right, and ready to sin again."

He laughed and insisted, "No, I'm serious. Will I be one hundred per cent cured?"

They do not want an ambiguous or jocular answer. They want certainty. But science, medical science, is only approximation. Certainty one should seek elsewhere.

108

He walked into my office, very dignified, fortyish. On his island in the West Indies he could be a teacher or perhaps a clergyman. He spoke English well enough and understood it even better, but he sported the usual hesitations with which people who have suffered a lot from officialdom try to gain time.

"Are you allergic to penicillin?"

"Yes, oh, yes!" But then he recovered himself. "No, I'm not allergic to penicillin."

"So you've had penicillin on your island and it didn't affect you badly?"

He nodded.

"Have you ever had a venereal disease?"

"No," he answered with conviction. "I had syphilis, but I never had venereal disease." Such faulty communication makes life difficult for a doctor. I only wonder what errors are made in police stations and in courts for the same reason.

Why do they come here with their chancres and claps, their inflamed ovaries and testicles? Can't they stay on their islands, and we'll send them the needed money and equipment? Often we feel this way (but we don't say it).

Once, a patient whom I refused to treat because he had no symptoms of any venereal disease whatsoever threatened noisily to complain to the supervisor. He got this answer from me (through an interpreter): "I, too, have a complaint to lodge: why doesn't he learn English if he has been here for two years and takes advantage of all our services?"

109

This boy of eighteen had a positive Dark Field. At that stage, syphilis is very contagious. He had to go to see the investigator on another floor, and to make sure that he would not disappear, I sent two young girls, student lab technicians, along with him. They each took the boy by one hand and, laughing and joking as youngsters will, led him away.

Afterward I asked the girls, "Didn't you feel squeamish about taking him by the hand?"

"No," they said, very surprised and still happily smiling, "not at all."

110

The heavy-set, middle-aged Puerto Rican explained that he had already gone to two doctors and they had cheated him. He wanted a real shot of penicillin. He wanted to be cured! I gave him the real shot. He reached into his pocket, brought out a ten-dollar bill, and handed it to me.

"Please, Doctor, I know you are a good doctor. Please take this for yourself."

I thanked him, refused politely, and advised him to give some poor man in the street a dollar.

Later, I was driving to another clinic. At a red light, a smiling, almost translucent Negro youth came up to my window and said, "For God's sake, man, give me a dollar. You can save me." And he smiled what impressed me as an angelic smile. I gave him a quarter.

"What kind of people are you?" he yelled in a rage, and I realized that his smile had been a painful grimace, a sort of tic. "I need a dollar and you give me a quarter! Look at my hands. They're all swollen. I must get to a hospital. . . ."

The light had changed, but I looked at his hands and arms. Punctured with injections, old and new, they were indeed inflamed and swollen.

"I need a dollar, too," I said, and stepped on the gas.

111

The boy didn't know a word of English but had found his way here from Greece. After delicately explaining to him in gestures that he had to drop his pants and show his genitals, I easily determined that he had gonorrhea.

"Are you allergic to penicillin? *Alérgico a la penicilina Usted?*" I was trying to get through to him in every possible way. He only smiled humbly and, when I became impatient, answered a vague "Yes," immediately followed by a "No," trying to appease me.

As it happens, we have a Greek bacteriologist, but that day he had chosen to stay away from the job. So I called his home. His mother, who answered the phone, consented to speak to the boy and, after a rather lengthy interchange, reported that "This is a very nice boy; I know the island he comes from."

"Is he allergic to penicillin?"

"He says he never had penicillin." That was good enough for me.

My colleague, who was giving the treatments that day, could not understand why the boy acted so dumb. "No speak English," I explained.

The doctor, an elderly man with an eternal cigar and a cough, suddenly got agitated.

"How can they go to bed with a woman if they don't know the language?" he asked irately.

"They speak an international language," the nurse said.

"I didn't know there was such a tongue," the doctor said peevishly. "I should have learned it, too."

"And now it's too late," said the nurse.

While all this was going on, the youth, his pants down and smiling his ancient Greek smile, watched us, like a thoroughbred dog in the veterinarian's office.

112

"If you made this patient S 47, you shouldn't have treated him," said the physician in charge, smiling peacefully. He has been on the job since 1939 and has long ago come to the conclusion that the only way to take it is to take it easy.

This particular boy had been brought in as a contact of a patient of ours who was under treatment for syphilis. Technically he should have been classified S 90 and received preventive treatment. But I found out that, three years before, he had had syphilis on his own and was treated for it. That made him S 47. But by making him S 47 I had lost the grounds for a treatment now.

"Why don't you make him S 40?" said the chief, smiling again peacefully but also shrewdly. S 40 stands for old, inadequately treated syphilis—which gives the right to inject penicillin.

This is how the hair is split in contemporary scientific conclaves. The cardinals who, in the Middle Ages, debated how many angels can stand on the point of a needle have nothing on us. They had to beware of the Holy Inquisition; we have to watch out for the Central Office.

113

The Greek came in with the manners of a man of the world: one who has been around. And indeed, he had been around; as a sailor with the merchant marine he had doubled both Capes several times. He was born on one of the Aegean islands; I couldn't make out whether he still owned a house there, whether he had sold it or wanted to sell it. And, of course, he had had several gonorrheas, "Ha, ha, ha." And was not allergic to penicillin, "Ha ha, ha." He certainly felt at ease in my office.

I processed him and gave him the routine shots. He was grateful and civil, and we had a nice chat about his island and real-estate possibilities there.

A while later, when I went to my locker to change, I found, in that little, closetlike room, my Greek in the company of three young girls. Idealistic student nurses from the Health Department, they had initiated a service of information and indoctrination (enlightening and propaganda) for patients with gonorrhea, similar to the one the investigators carry on for syphilitics.

It was with this purpose that they had locked themselves up with the Greek sailor and, surrounded by pamphlets, colored pictures, and textbooks, were lecturing him.

When I entered the room, the girls fell silent, waiting for me to leave. My presence embarrassed them. But Ulysses, his face sweating, his eyes shining, gave me a wink: he was having the time of his life.

Instead of answering my introductory question about penicillin, he said, "May I explain something to you, Doctor, sir?
I do not speak well English, and you have to give me time
to speak correctly."

"Okay. Shoot."

"My father and mother had syphilis." He pronounced
the *sy* as in "cyclon."

"Yes?" I encouraged him.

"When I was three years old they found that I had cyphilis,
too, and had me treated by a doctor."

"How old are you now?"

"Twenty-seven."

"And what brings you here today?"

"I want to know whether my blood is good."

"Fine. We'll take a sample and you'll come in a week for
the result."

"Is it safe for me to wait a whole week?"

"You waited twenty-four years and now you're making a
fuss over one week!"

He was silent for a moment, as if chewing on my words;
then, looking belligerent, he consented. I cleaned his skin
with an alcohol sponge, stuck in the needle, withdrew 5 c.c.
of blood, and was about to apply the same sponge again
when he stopped me.

"You dropped this cotton on the floor and now you put
it on my wound!"

"I never dropped it on the floor. It was here, on the table."

"Excuse me, I meant to say that you dropped this cotton
on the table and now it's not clean."

"You're a bore, you know. It's all over. Go into the next
room."

"I'm not a bore," he said, with a malignant grimace. "It's

my health. I have to protect it. You don't give a damn about me."

"For twenty-four years you protected yourself, and look at the results!" I showed him the cotton, which was soot-black—the fellow apparently hadn't washed for the last twenty-four years. He walked out, giving me another hate-filled glance.

115

The handsome, intelligent-looking Negro boy of seventeen had come with a fresh case of gonorrhea. His chart showed that it was the third gonorrhea in two years. He refused the injections. He wanted pills.

"Why?" I asked.

"Because I'm afraid."

"If you aren't afraid to pick up strange girls in the street, you shouldn't be afraid of a needle."

He considered himself offended. "I'll complain to your superior!" he murmured unconvincingly.

"Give him the pills and get him out of here," I told the nurse. I thought that I was through with him, but half an hour later I noticed him following me from one end of the hall to the other. Finally he said, "Please, Doctor, don't get mad. Tell me, what's the difference between pills and needles?"

"The injection is stronger. It cured you twice before. For you it's a sure thing."

"But I'm afraid of the needle."

"Where is your pride?" I said. "Are you a man or a mouse?"

"It's not a question of pride. It's a question of pain. Pride I've got, but pain I can't stand."

"We are here in life to stand some pain, too. Didn't they tell you that in school, in church, in the movies?"

"No, they didn't."

"What books do you read in school?" I asked.

He thought for quite a while and then hesitantly answered, "Hawthorne . . ."

116

Another boy of seventeen.

"I bet you picked her up on the street."

"No," he exclaimed, lighting up in a smile. "I've known her all my life. We grew up on the same block."

"Well, she's not a nice girl any more," I interjected. "She gave you a bad disease."

"Oh, yes, she is nice! She didn't always have it. She got it from someone else."

"Yes," I confirmed, "you are right: she got it from someone else."

He seemed satisfied, even happy.

117

He is twenty-four. White and smart. An architect, he says. This is his fourth gonorrhea in a year.

"Would you know from whom you got it? Could you send this person in to get treated, too?"

"How long does it take to develop a fresh gonorrhea?" he asked coolly.

"From one day to a week."

"A whole week? No, I wouldn't know who it was," he answered promptly, and smiled. Cool, smart. While zipping up his pants, he said very self-assuredly, "Doctor, I meant to ask you: who had the first V.D., a man or a woman?"

"Well, which came first, the egg or the chicken?" I challenged him.

"Oh," he said, "it's one of those questions, is it?" And he lost interest in the conversation.

"Tell me, how is your math?" I inquired.

"Math?" He was so surprised that his air of coolness faded away.

"Yes, math. Doesn't an architect need a lot of math?"

"No, I don't believe so." Again, with much superiority, "I'm an artist."

118

He was in his thirties. No longer young, as far as our clients go, and a real bore.

"You don't have gonorrhea," I had repeated several times. But he kept nagging me.

"Seems impossible. She told me she had it. And I stayed with her all night."

"Where was that?"

"In Florida."

"Did you know her before?"

"No, it was a sort of vacation. Could it be, Doctor," he continued, "that she invented it to scare me off, to get rid of me?"

"I don't know." I didn't want to hurt his feelings. But really, I wouldn't blame her. . . .

"Do women often use this as a pretext?" he kept on, apparently lost on unfamiliar territory.

"No, I don't think so. It is a rather degrading thing to admit to. In such a case a woman usually says that she's having her period."

"What is a period?" he asked, with a hungry spark in his eyes.

Nervous, excited, very good-looking (professionally good-looking: a gambler, a gigolo), he told me a complicated story.

He is supposed to appear in court today. A month ago, a doctor had diagnosed syphilis and given him pills, which he has been taking ever since. Proof: two empty boxes with labels from a pharmacy. Now he wants a letter for the judge, stating that he is under treatment, so that his case can be put off until he is completely cured.

Why doesn't his private doctor give him the letter? This he could not explain. We offered to take a blood test and, should further treatment be necessary, to administer it. But he didn't want a test.

"I need that letter today," he said, "not in a week." And, very dissatisfied with us, he rushed out, probably to another clinic.

We have a new investigator. Fresh from training, well-groomed, serious, and pleasant-looking, with no FBI airs or pretensions about him.

"How do you conduct an investigation?" I ask him.

"You mean, how do we handle a new case?"

"Yes. Let's assume a fellow walks in with a primary syphilis. How do you go about his contacts? I assume that's what is most important, isn't it? Suppose he refuses to give any information? Does that happen?"

"Yes, quite often."

"What is the reason for such refusals?"

"Mostly private reasons. They are afraid the family—their parents, wife, children—will become aware of the episode."

"So what do you do?"

"It's important to reassure them that their privacy will be protected. That under no circumstances will their name be divulged to other parties. You use fear and motivation," he said, proud of his recently acquired scientific vocabulary.

"What is your background?" I ask him. "Did you go to college?"

"Yes, I have a B.A."

"And how long did this special course take?"

"One month."

"What do they mean by fear and motivation?"

"You tell him that the other party will sooner or later get caught and then report his name as a contact. Which means that the investigator will visit his home, write, or call him. That frightens them. And of course there is the moral approach: to help us check the disease! You have to lie a bit, tell him that, if he previously had penicillin, syphilis will not show up on him in the usual way. That's scary, too. And you explain that he's not doing anything wrong by mentioning other people's names. The idea is to eradicate this dreadful disease, and then it will be safe for everybody to make love and be happy. No publicity, strict privacy, hygiene, and science!"

"Suppose he honestly doesn't know the origin, that first party from whom he caught it?"

"That seldom happens. Only if it was a prostitute or a pickup, a homosexual from a Turkish bath."

"A Turkish bath!" I was surprised. I hadn't known about this aspect of the Turkish bath.

"Oh, yes, that's where homosexuals go for contacts. It's the easiest and most dangerous place."

"Do they have the opportunity and the space to make love there? In these miserable establishments?" Somehow I couldn't believe it.

"Of course they do."

91

"And what about such cases? Is it hopeless to pursue them?"

"Not really. If you know the neighborhood where the prostitute was picked up or the bar or the Turkish bath, you can net several possibilities at once and process them until you find the one that is infected. To hold people for a day or so and then let them back onto the streets makes sense. We get a blood test, and afterward we follow them up."

This young, neat, agreeable investigator wants to get his Ph.D. in sociology. But that calls for work, and he can't give up his income, especially now that jobs are scarce. And besides, being an investigator is exciting, at least in the beginning.

121

The Parisian, a blonde with fair skin and slightly red pubic hair, was neither beautiful nor elegant, but her genitals were kept in such shining condition that it was clear: love (or rather, making love) was her vocation!

She had come to New York on a tourist visa but would like to remain for good. "I'm twenty-five," she said, and this was probably not more than six or seven years short of the truth.

Her cervix, although in no way inflamed, was thick and dilated.

"Have you had any children?" I asked.

"*Mais non, monsieur*," she answered indignantly, "I'm not married."

The investigator and the bacteriologist, both young fellows, stood behind the plastic screen, listening to our French conversation, their faces reflecting exotic visions.

"Yes," I told them afterward, "that was a real Parisian!"

They nodded, and smiled dreamily.

122

He showed up again. Once a week he comes to pester me. Circassian or Iranian, from a village near the Caspian Sea. He is dripping, but we can't find any trace of gonorrhea in his discharge. Therefore he does not belong in a V.D. clinic; he should go to the genitourinary division of a hospital.

However, he chooses to pester me and, every time, begs for a shot of penicillin. He wears a long, thick (pornographic) mustache, and when he begins to bring out his huge sexual machine with the two distinctly oversized testicles, his face assumes a ritualistic, wild expression, as if he were drawing a sacred dagger from a bejeweled ancient scabbard.

Afterward he elegantly, with a specific Asian grace, zips himself up and, stepping noiselessly on his soft rubber soles, walks out—obviously irresistible to the women of his tribe.

123

The men's toilet is worth mentioning. In short, it's filthy. Filthy, although once a day a man in heavy-duty gloves goes in and cleans it. It can't be kept clean. Especially since there is a trick for flushing: you have to press down hard (best with your foot) and wait for a long moment; only then does it begin to drain. If you don't press long enough, nothing happens.

I have devised a complicated and, I hope, foolproof technique for using this necessary commodity. First, while still in the working room, I wash my hands. Then I take a paper towel, and, protecting my hands with it, I open the door and close it the same way. Then I take a fresh paper towel and approach the toilet (there are no urinals), which is filled up with the usual things plus paper and cigarette butts. From the wall directly to the left a huge inscription greets me: WATCH OUT: THIS COULD BE A CLAPTRAP! Underneath, several appropriate commentaries (they change).

After every step in my adventure I reach for a fresh paper towel; walking out, I again use a new one, still protecting myself from the contaminated knobs. Back in my office I wash my hands. I would advise every customer of ours to adopt this routine; it is a pity we have no pamphlet on the subject.

Of course, there is a separate washroom for the doctors and laboratory technicians, with a special key attached to a huge wooden board and kept under lock in a special drawer. But I don't bother. And, after all, why should the knobs in there be less contaminated?

124

"Doctor, how long does it take for clap to develop?" He was slim, very fair, barely twenty.

"Why? Do you want to figure out who gave it to you?"

"Yes, I'd like to."

"From one day to one week," I said.

"It couldn't be a month?" he asked, disappointed.

"No, not according to the old textbooks. Did you want to exempt one particular person?"

"Yes, I did," he whispered, looking really sad.

125

He is going off to report for a newspaper on the European summer festivals and would like a blood test before leaving.

"Doctor," he said, "I just got my vaccination. Does it look

right to you?" He showed me an acutely positive smallpox vaccination.

"It looks as if you needed it," I said. "But I wouldn't advise you to check on your blood right now. The vaccination may distort your immunological reactions."

He could not grasp this. "What difference does it make?"

"It may interfere with the results of the test, and for the rest of your life you might remain under the impression that you were once positive for syphilis. Psychologically that is hard to shake off."

"Oh, psychologically," he said condescendingly. "I don't care. Take my blood."

126

On Ninth Avenue there is a church, basically Episcopal but with a strange inscription on the side: Orthodox American. Since I pass this way twice a week, I often enter through the inviting portals, sit for a while, look at the stained-glass windows, and listen to the silence, characteristic of churches and cemeteries between the acts.

Sometimes a tall, middle-aged Negro, perching close to the ceiling on a high ladder, putters around the chandeliers. He looks at me, I look at him, we both are silent; the entire scene may be interpreted as an illustration to a work by Kafka. There is definitely tension between us. How can I convince him that I don't want to steal the silver or commit some sacrilege?

One day I chanced there upon the "wedding" of two boys. It was then that I realized that I had strayed into the church for homosexuals about which I had read in the *New York Times*. Over 100 men and women had gathered to witness the new sacrament. Some faces were familiar, and one man even greeted me.

"How do you like it?" he asked, with obvious partisan interest.

"I really don't know. How do you feel about it?"

"Well, it gives us status. I like it." And he repeated very firmly, "I like it."

127

"Why were there so many cases of epidemiological syphilis today?" I asked the chief.

"Last week we had several positive Dark Fields, so the investigators combed the neighborhood for contacts." Those who have been in contact with a fresh syphilis, we classify as S 90 and immediately give them their first shot of penicillin. A strong shot!

Yesterday two of my patients collapsed after the injection. The first one—a weakling studying psychology at a teachers' college—probably fainted at the sight of the thick needle. I had to lift this six-footer up and lay him out flat on the table. Before I realized that this was not an allergic reaction, I had my moments of agony, and for this, of course, I hold a grudge against him.

The second manifested the typical picture of anaphylactic shock. I had to inject Adrenalin and cortisone and feed him oxygen before he came to and his pulse and respiration straightened out.

All this because of a massive dose of penicillin, which possibly he did not need: he denied having had any contact with our patient. But whom are we to believe?

128

Two boys, ex-addicts, sent to us by a rehabilitation center called The Compass, for a routine checkup on V.D.

"How do you like The Compass?"

"I like it," said one.

"I like it very much," said the second.

"What treatment do they give you?"

"Group therapy," said the first.

"They help us to understand why we are the way we are," answered the second.

That one was nineteen; the other, fourteen.

"What do you think of methadone?" I put my usual question.

They did not like it. "That's not for young people. It's another kind of addiction," they both agreed. "For older ones it's okay."

129

A boy of nineteen, sent to us for a checkup by the psychiatric division of one of the city courts.

"What's wrong with you, son?" was my question.

"Nothing is wrong with me. It's four years now that I've been trying to shake off this charge."

"What is the charge?"

"They say I cut him up with a knife. I never touched him, and they have no proof."

"And why are you in the psychiatric division?"

"I don't know. My lawyer . . ."

"I hope you'll be all right," I said. "Next time don't use a knife."

"I didn't use a knife," he corrected me, and winked discreetly.

How much more intelligent than the other half of humanity these delinquents, derelicts, and addicts often are! And what a wonderful capacity for jokes! Is it an accident that their opposite numbers in the Health Department, the courts, and the police force are completely devoid of any sense of humor?

130

He arrived in a state of great agitation. A huge, obese man in his middle thirties. Last Friday he went with a prostitute.

"I didn't have sex with her. She only goofed around my prick," he explained. But now the inside of his mouth and his tongue are swollen and itchy.

"You must be the nervous type," I said. "After all, she goofed around you; you didn't goof around her."

"I, too, kissed her and stuck my tongue inside her mouth."

"Do you have any other symptoms? Sores, rashes?"

"No. You see, Doctor, I want to be ahead of those signs. If my wife notices anything, she'll leave me. You understand. She already says that I'm too fat."

"You don't want her to leave you?"

"No. We've been married three years and I went only twice with other women. You know how it is."

His face was huge, asymmetrical, greasy. His eyes were sharp and on the defensive, constantly expecting danger from every corner.

"Were you ever in a state hospital?" I asked.

"Yes, I was. It's where I met my wife. That's why I can't reason with her."

"Do you have children?"

"No, we tried. But we don't have any," he said apologetically.

"What's your profession, your trade?"

"I'm a messenger now."

"Come back in a week and I'll tell you the result of the test. The way I see it, you don't have V.D. However, since you are so sensitive, I'd advise you to stay away from prostitutes. You know how it is. . . ." I kicked back to him that stupid sentence that our patients throw at us all day long in an attempt to justify the most absurd situations.

131

He came in, bringing the smell of alcohol and of the Bowery with him. Indeed, he was pleasantly drunk, smiling and stuttering. And there was a deep laceration on his nose. He was a Negro in his thirties.

He had had syphilis long ago, but now he had gonorrhea, and a big ulcer on his leg was bothering him (I had never seen such an ulcer except on the *clochards* of Paris). Actually, this time he did not want treatment but a letter for the Welfare Department, confirming that he was sick and needed continuation of relief. (For some reason they had dropped him from the rolls.) I could not issue such a letter. We argued for a while about this until screams and noises from the next room caused us to rush there together.

We have a special kind of penicillin for gonorrhea: it is very strong and very soluble, *i.e.*, it enters and is absorbed by the organism very quickly. This is the reason why many patients pass out right after receiving the injection. It so happened that one of our doctors had just administered this particular kind of penicillin and the patient had collapsed. When I rushed into the room, he was clinging to the wall and slowly sliding down, his body stiff, his face expressionless, looking just like Buster Keaton. I grabbed him and tried to lift him up and carry him to the table. No one helped me. The doctor who had given the injection, an elderly man with a puffed-up, bluish face and a constant cough, was sitting on a chair, himself on the verge of fainting. The nurses were frozen to their stations. It was the drunkard with the lacerated nose who came to my help. Together we carried Buster Keaton to the table and put him down comfortably. Then I took care of him, of his tongue that was wedged between his teeth, of his slowing pulse. Adrenalin and cortisone did the trick; he slowly came to and even began to speak English, which, before, he had claimed not to understand. Only his knees remained wobbly; he could not stand up. We had to call an ambulance and transfer him to a hospital.

Later I saw my drunkard talking to the chief, trying to persuade him to sign a letter for the Welfare Department. (But chiefs don't like to sign such letters.)

I walked up to the man and shook his hand.

"You are the only one who helped when we needed it," I said. "You are a good sport."

He smiled magnanimously, like a king, and, speaking now much more firmly since the alcohol vapors had begun to dissipate, said, "Don't mention it, man."

132

He is a Hungarian refugee. Saturday night he went with a woman ("You know how it is"), and now he feels a burning pain when he urinates—exactly like fifteen years ago in Budapest.

"I know I got it," he assured me, trying to make light of it but actually very bitter. "She was a whore. I'm ashamed of myself."

There were no gonococci in his smear, and I gave him some pills to help his nonspecific urethritis. He thanked me profusely. He knew three or four words of Russian, and we exchanged them with friendly smiles.

Why all these men are so disgusted in retrospect with

their Saturday-night dates is a puzzle to me. They call them whores even if they are not whores, and they never seem to recall how attracted they were by these "whores" only a few nights ago. Women are less treacherous. They are perhaps not so strongly attracted right away, but later they don't complain as much, either.

133

He was fifteen. A black.

"Do you know who gave it to you?"

"No," he answered after a moment of hard thinking. "There were two girls."

"Why do you need two girls at the same time?" I asked.

"It wasn't at the same time," he said, obviously refraining from adding something like "idiot."

I processed him as quickly as possible.

"You're very rough," he complained after the injections.

"You should thank me, not complain, you idiot," I said. At the end of a day, with all those ingrates and ignoramuses, your nerves are on edge.

The boy didn't react to my remark. But later, before leaving for the street, he stuck his head into my room and said, "Thank you!" It made quite a difference.

134

A doctor in his seventies, who had gone through a brain hemorrhage and was still partially paralyzed, got a job with us. Both his hands were shaking, half his face was an immobile mask, and he walked unsteadily. We all wanted to be helpful: apparently his so-called Social Security was not enough for him to live on. He only gave injections, a technical performance of which he was quite capable. But his hands were shaky and his speech was stumbling, and one of the cruel and always-right customers complained. In the middle of a session, he was sent home.

His face a pale mask, his gait a mixture of drag and jump, he looked at us with unseeing eyes and silently shuffled out of our lives, forever.

135

You can't moralize with our young patients. You can't talk to them about Western civilization, the church, or education, for all these are parts of the establishment and responsible for the mess we are in. But they are not down on all religion. They like to hear about Hindu practices, Far Eastern rites, Yoga technique. These have nothing to do with our police or politics and are somehow connected with science, with deep breathing, gymnastics, hygiene, meditation, fresh air, ecology.

It is pathetic how these young people, ready to blow up the entire establishment, revere science, which is so important a part of it. Herein lies their greatest contradiction: "Culture, *no!* Penicillin, *sí!*"

As for Christianity, it has left a bitter taste in their mouths. It will take decades of *aggiornamenti*, imprisoned radical priests and nuns, to eradicate the ambiguous historical memories.

136

"It means that you went with the wrong woman."

He laughed the laughter of a healthy twenty-two-year-old charmer. "Have you ever seen the right woman?" he retorted.

"Do you believe women are worse than men?"

"I do believe that," he said firmly.

"In what respect, morally or intellectually?"

"They lie more," he replied without hesitation.

"Don't men lie?" I asked.

"Yes, of course, but not really. Because everybody knows they aren't telling the truth."

He zipped up his pants and vanished into Central Harlem, a successful Casanova.

137

"In spite of all the treatments it keeps coming back. So I figured maybe it's my girl friend who has it and should be under care."

"Very smart of you," I encouraged him. "How long have you been sleeping with her?"

"Two months. And we don't fool around."

"That's nice. How old is she?"

"Eighteen."

"And you?'

"Thirty."

They both had gonorrhea, and after the injections they left together. He put an arm around her hips: a sign of exclusive possession, warning the other males to keep off. She looked very young, with firm breasts and smooth, tanned legs. They smiled at each other, thus publicly confirming their happiness, and walked through the large hall, obviously in love (whatever that may mean).

138

He is twenty-two. He was once treated for an acquired syphilis and has a long history of gonorrheas. Now he has come again, "dripping."

When I saw his veins I said, "You take heroin."

"Not any more; I used to."

"How did you straighten out?"

"It was easy," he said. "I wasn't really hooked."

"How does one know whether one is hooked or not?"

"I couldn't tell at the time," he explained. "You do know, though, later."

139

She had well-defined veins, but when I hit one with the needle, no blood came. The vein was atrophied.

"Why didn't you tell me that you inject the stuff?" I complained.

She giggled. "I wanted you to find out for yourself."

She was very short, under five feet, and very pale; quite an ugly little thing. What man would go for her? But apparently she had found at least one.

"You should bring in your boy friend," I suggested. "We'll treat him, too."

"He's gone to Boston," she said, smiling tenderly. "He'll see a private doctor. No"—she stopped me—"those veins are no good. Try here!" She rotated her forearm and abandoned it to me with an innocent, dreamy, somewhat lewd smile, as if she were making me a proposition.

She was small, pale, and ugly, and yet there was something

in her that made her important, if not dangerous. So does a miserable alley cat have traits in common with the royal tiger.

140

The two women had come together: a couple, gone to seed, pitiful. I have seen many such creatures in Europe; I have not met them much in New York. Both were junkies; both had sores in their vaginas. One of them kept speaking about her husband, not saying much, however, except that there *was* a husband. The other, at 10 A.M., smelled of liquor. She wanted a drink of water and kept asking for the fountain and the paper cups.

Now, the sad fact is that our fountain doesn't work, and paper cups are not always to be found. Millions of dollars are spent on the strongest, speediest antibiotics, on disposable syringes and undisposable, but useless, clerks and aides, but the Board of Health can't afford a clean gown once a week for a doctor, let alone paper cups. We could perhaps afford these things if it were not that special personnel would be needed to handle them. The VIPs stay in the office and never venture into the jungle of their departments. So they don't really know what's going on there—except from memos and circulars.

I took the patient to the pantry (right across from the women's treatment room, where all the refuse from their leaking organs is gradually accumulated in the course of the day). There the nurses make coffee for themselves and some of the doctors. Since I very soon lost my taste for coffee there, I was glad to lend my cup to thirsty or faint patients.

"Here's some water," I said to this drunken fallen angel with the many sores. "I don't drink here. When I'm thirsty I go to the bar on the next block." It was supposed to be a joke, but she took it seriously.

105

"Oh. And do you speak to the women there?" Suddenly she looked at me with professional interest. The mention of the bar (next block) made me human and open to suggestions.

141

"I'm ashamed of myself. . . ."

That is a familiar opening for some men. Last Saturday he was drunk, and a pack of young fellows jumped and raped him.

"My ass is burning and leaking."

He was in his early forties, very masculine, athletic, and didn't look like a bum. What had happened to him was an accident.

"Professionals" don't excuse themselves, don't mention rape. They are very matter-of-fact and *demand* a checkup on both anus and penis, as if they paid double taxes. Some even come regularly twice a month without any symptoms.

"Anything wrong about checking?" they ask belligerently. "That's what you're getting paid for, isn't it?"

142

She looked as if any moment she might break into tears. She was slim, in blue jeans and a denim jacket.

"Twenty-two?"

"No, I'm nineteen."

"What's your complaint?"

"I don't know how to put it to you. You see, all my girl friends made fun of me because I was still a virgin," she began, almost in a whisper.

"Yes, go on, silly," I said, to encourage her.

She smiled through wet eyes. "So last Thursday, at a party, I let him do it," she finished with relief.

"You met him there for the first time?"

"Yes."

"Will you see him again?"

"I don't know. I don't think so."

"Do you care about him?"

"No, not at all."

"So why did you do it, stupid?"

"Everybody made fun of me, and I really don't see any point in being a virgin. Besides, I had a couple of drinks."

"Was he drunk, too?"

"Yes," she said hesitantly. "He was drinking."

For young and old alike, this business of "having been drunk" is a sacramental excuse in our society for anything bad we want to do and would do anyway, even if booze had never been invented.

"And now of course you are afraid you caught V.D.?" I asked. First-timers usually expect V.D. and/or a baby right away.

"Yes," she explained, "it hurts."

"Did you bleed much?"

"No," she said with surprise, "very little. But I feel something like a sore there."

I put in a speculum to examine her. We have only two sizes and the smaller is still too large for such a patient. In short, she moaned and cried and, at the end of the examination, began to bleed. Obviously the hymen had not been completely torn, and my speculum finished the job.

"You should watch your next period," I told her. "If it's late you'd better go to a gynecologist."

"He said he took precautions," she explained, still on the table, her legs spread and her eyes wet.

"What kind of precautions?"

"He pulled it out," she said, looking at me interrogatively.

"Did he tell you that?" I asked.

107

"No, he told my roommate. She called him up. But I guess this isn't too sure, is it?"

"No, it isn't sure," said the nurse, who apparently knew what she was talking about. "Move back and get up!"

143

The girl, a Puerto Rican with frank breasts and smooth skin, small but a perfect woman at eighteen, smiled like a child. Apparently she was a sweet, good girl.

"Do you speak English?" I asked. Such a happy, innocent look usually goes with "no speak English."

She laughed and said good-naturedly, "Of course I speak English."

"What's the problem?"

The story was a short one: her mother had syphilis and so the girl wanted to check on her blood, too. It made sense. I took a blood sample and told her to wait outside until a table was free for a vaginal examination. Meanwhile I called in the next patient, a small Puerto Rican woman in her late forties, "no speak English." That can be an agony.

I had the brilliant idea of using the previous patient— the fresh, innocent, smiling girl—as interpreter. I called her in.

"Please ask her whether she is allergic to penicillin," I said.

The girl, smiling her best, most courteous smile, pronounced four or five sentences in which the word *alérgica* figured prominently. And the middle-aged woman, smiling sheepishly, answered, "No. No alérgica."

"Ask her why she came here."

Without losing time, the girl answered, "She has syphilis and came to have a checkup and to be treated."

Only then did it dawn upon me that these were mother and daughter, who had come together to the clinic.

There is a short story by Tchekhov. . . . It takes place in court. At a critical moment the defendant, in order to get support for his statement, appeals to the guard to confirm it. Whereupon it turns out that the guard is the prisoner's son. The judge, the prosecutor, and all present are stupefied by this coincidence. I received something of a similar shock when I suddenly realized the relationship between the two women.

However, since we were already in midstream, I chose to go on. The daughter told me that a year ago her mother had acquired a lover who turned out to have syphilis, and six months ago the woman was treated at New York Hospital. Whether the lover was ever treated they did not know. Now the girl's fiancé insisted on a checkup for both of them.

To my delight, this intimate talk drew mother and daughter closer together. Hand in hand they walked out of my office and, outside, sitting on the bench, kept up a peaceful conversation.

Incidentally, when I sent the girl out while I examined the mother on the table, the latter suddenly began to understand English quite well and to express herself without any need of an interpreter.

"How come you don't know whether your lover was ever treated for syphilis?" I asked. It really puzzled me. But she did not find it strange.

"I never asked him," she said.

144

"Last Saturday . . ." They often start with those words: last Saturday, last Friday, last Tuesday. Apparently the notion of time is important.

Last Saturday, ran his trite story, he went to a bar, a sort of neighborhood club, where he met a woman. And now he is dripping.

He was a simple, healthy-looking boy, with bushy hair. Such a fellow would take his shots easily and probably be cured in a week or so.

But his story had a complicated angle. His girl friend had gone home to Jamaica on a vacation and was coming back Sunday. Would he be able to meet her expectations Sunday night without danger of infecting her?

"No, you must wait an entire week. Then we'll check again for gonorrhea, and we'll also have the results of your blood test," I explained in a neutral voice. (I do it fifty times a day.)

"But that's impossible," he exclaimed in real anguish. "She'll guess that something's wrong."

"Do you care a lot about her?" I asked.

"Yes."

"Then tell her the truth," I said.

For a moment he was taken aback, then he smiled, nodded his bushy head energetically, and walked out with a resolute air.

145

What a day! We had about fifteen cases of contact syphilis, and all of them, whether they had symptoms or not, were given the first shot of penicillin. It's a lot of work and mostly useless, since the results of the blood test are only known a week later.

One of these fellows collapsed. He had a genuine allergic shock, which we managed to control with Adrenalin, cortisone, and oxygen. With sixty or seventy patients sitting side by side on the benches this is quite a dramatic spectacle. The questions arise again and again in my mind whether we should so casually administer these horse doses of penicillin; whether Social Hygiene isn't perhaps in contradiction with the interests of the individual.

A second patient, too, passed out. But he was simply one

of those who can't stand the pointed, thick needle and the sight of their own blood. A whiff of ammonia promptly brought him around. He was an Italian who barely spoke English and who now, under the influence of the shock, began to implore me in French, *"Parle-moi français, parle-moi français!"*

For half an hour I had to talk to him in French, telling him over and over that he was all right, that he shouldn't get panicky, that there was nothing wrong with his heart. (He claimed his father had died young from a heart attack.) The moment I stopped and was about to walk away from him, he started to writhe and to yell, *"Parle-moi français, parle-moi français!"* He wanted undivided attention, this spoiled, good-for-nothing twenty-two-year-old—who was already on his seventh gonorrhea, all of them different strains from different countries. Last year, in Switzerland, he had nearly died in a doctor's office, he told me. *"Parle-moi français, parle-moi français!"* What he was doing in the United States I didn't find out and I couldn't have cared less.

"Oui, oui, ce sont vos nerfs. Calmez-vous donc. Vous avez une blennorragie; ce n'est rien," I shouted. *"Ce n'est qu'une chaudepisse."*

But this did not satisfy him, and he kept coming back at me with his *"Parle-moi français, parle-moi français!"*

To finish the day, an epileptic found it appropriate to throw a fit while I was taking a sample of his blood. He was a little man from Harlem, with an asymmetrical skull and an infected ass. I wonder whether he sometimes has his attacks in bed underneath another guy.

Accidents like these usually come in clusters. There are days when nothing untoward occurs, but once a knot has formed in the skein it somehow sets up a chain reaction. As things were, I was grateful that I hadn't given the epileptic penicillin, for probably I shouldn't have been able to distinguish his attack from an anaphylactic shock. To get a comprehensible past history from our patients is practically impossible.

111

He was standing with his back toward me, expecting his shot of penicillin.

"Let your pants down," I reminded him.

He did, displaying a white, average-looking behind.

"What are you studying?" I asked, to distract him from the needle.

"Oh . . . political science."

"Here is a good topic for your future thesis: the influence of V.D. on politics," I said, to distract him from the second shot.

"Maybe it's a good topic," he answered brusquely, "but it won't bring me any money."

It was then I noticed that not only his buttocks but everything about him was average and boring.

147

Some people are born with deformed arms or legs. Whether it is due to a medication the mother took during pregnancy or to a virus infection such as German measles is beside the point here. Many factors can interfere with the normal growth of a fetus (only thoughts, it seems, don't cripple).

He was born with shaved-off fingers. Imagine a heavy, well-built Negro boy growing up in Harlem without fingers.

"You just can't take enough precautions," he said, when I told him that he had gonorrhea. I wondered what kind of precautions he did take, and how he performed, without his hands to guide him.

"Yessir!" I agreed. "And how much did it cost you?"

He thought for a moment and amiably answered, "All in all, eight dollars."

"Eight dollars!" I exaggerated my surprise. "What can you expect for eight dollars these days?"

He laughed and then said, "Yes, the dollar isn't what it used to be."

148

"What bullshit," he said, in answer to my remark about the exorbitant price of heroin. "A shot of the stuff costs three or four dollars, five at the most. They tell you lies in the papers. I pay five dollars for the best stuff, believe me."

He is a cook; hard-working, twenty-two years old. He makes a good living. On Sundays he indulges himself with one or two shots of heroin. "It relaxes me. Why not? I'm not hooked." Now he has contracted syphilis. But we'll cure him, of course. . . .

The preponderance of V.D. among junkies is striking. To the best of my knowledge, no reliable statistics are available, and the picture is further complicated by the fact that the use of heroin interferes with the normal serological reaction of the blood, thus giving many junkies a positive reaction for syphilis even if they don't have it. So there is still a lot to be explored, and common sense would suggest a merger of drug and V.D. clinics. But our public services are miserably fragmented. Suffice it to say that infections of the ureter, prostate, and bladder due to so-called nonspecific urethritis, are completely removed from the V.D. clinics' jurisdiction. A woman may be in agony from a vaginal fungus (*Monilia*) or trichomoniasis, but she gets no help from us, because she has a disease classified as nonvenereal. A man may suffer from severe urethritis—but if it is not obviously caused by gonococci, we send him to another clinic.

149

"I got syphilis twenty-seven years ago and I can't get rid of it," he said.

"How old are you?"

"Forty."

"Bad luck. Where did you get it at thirteen? In South America?"

"No, right here in New York. . . . I'd like to know: am I the only one who can't be cured, or are there others like me?"

"You aren't the only one who keeps showing a positive reaction."

This statement really seemed to relieve and console him.

150

She had come—on her day off—all the way from Bridgeport, Connecticut. A month ago she had noticed a heavy discharge. She went to a local physician, who gave her a shot of penicillin but did not take any tests. Now she had broken off with her boy friend and wanted to check again.

She was twenty, fair, with freckles, and her name was Cynthia. This had not been her first experience, but she was disappointed and had even given up the pill.

"What do you think of sex?" I asked to distract her. She was tense: biting her lips in expectation of the needle.

"It's all right, I guess," she answered without conviction.

"You have gonorrhea," I said. She looked blank. "Clap," I corrected myself.

"I see," she reacted. "I still occasionally meet this fellow. Should I tell him?"

"By all means," I said. "But many of them don't believe the woman. They claim she got it from someone else."

"Really?" Again she stiffened.

She reminded me of a character in a Dostoevski novel, an abused minor, poor and proud. I wanted to say something significant, something to help her go on, but didn't know what.

"You must look for durable things in life. There's no future for you in cold-blooded sex," I began.

"I have to go to the bathroom," she interrupted me. "Where is it, please?"

Here eyes were pale blue, the color of body secretions.

A week later she came for the results of the blood test, which were negative. Everything was negative now. The first injection had cured her. She was wearing a blue summer dress and red shoes and carrying a white pocketbook. There was something festive in her appearance.

It is striking how different they look when they first come for a checkup, and the second time, when they feel (in every cell) that they are cured.

151

Of the four doctors who were supposed to come that afternoon only one showed up: me. And I had a full house: eighty-five patients to see in two and a half hours.

In the middle of my struggle to clear the waiting room (a struggle in many ways reminiscent of driving crosstown from east to west through Manhattan) this little fairy appeared. He felt all right but wanted to be sure. Wasn't it a sound idea to have regular checkups?

"Yes, it's a good idea," I said wearily. "We'll take a blood sample for syphilis."

But the gay young man wasn't satisfied. He also wanted a rectal smear.

"For Christ's sake," I exploded, "don't you see how busy we are today with all the doctors away? And you come with your fucking ass for a routine checkup! Can't you postpone it until after Labor Day?"

"No," he said. "You're here to take care of us."

"And you, what do you do? Whom do you take care of?" I asked in a rage.

"I pay taxes," said this little bastard, who was probably on some kind of welfare. "And my father pays taxes. And all my family pays taxes."

I knew he was lying, but I couldn't prove it. And that wasn't the point, anyway.

152

She spread her legs, and in her pinkish skin, where short red hairs sprouted, a strawberry-red fissure came into view.

A woman philosopher and religious teacher of the fourth century, Hypatia of Alexandria, had a striking discussion with her lover. To discourage his earthly temptations, she addressed him, at the most passionate moment of their relations, in the following manner: "See what it is you adore, Archytas, this foul matter, this corruption, with its secretions, its excrements and its infections. . . ."

But the tenacious and passionate Archytas gave her this answer: "It is not matter I love, but form."

How many times, discouraged and depressed in the V.D. clinic, have I repeated these saintly words of Archytas . . .

"You were in contact with someone who has syphilis," I explained to him. I made a point of not specifying the sex, since I was not sure of my customer's tastes.

He cast an intense, almost cruel look at me.

"I'm at a loss, he said. "If you gave me some more details I might understand what you are talking about."

"It is really immaterial. We'll put you down for epidemiological syphilis and treat you preventively."

"I'm allergic to penicillin." He stopped me short.

In this situation smart old-timers pretend to such an allergy. We are in no position to doubt their statement, and in this way they escape shots which they consider superfluous.

"Very well," I said, "in that case we'll give you pills." Then I added, "You met this person on the . . . on the sixteenth of April." I am not supposed to use the investigator's data, but on and off I do, in order to get better cooperation.

"The sixteenth of April?" He became very businesslike. "Let me see." He extracted from his pocket a small address book filled with names and figures and quickly began to leaf through it. Something, however, apparently did not satisfy him. "Are you sure it was on the sixteenth?" he asked.

"That's what the report says," I confirmed.

In Paris, prostitutes of the better class used to carry such little books; at certain days and certain hours they had certain customers, listed well in advance for the entire month or, perhaps, year. I never knew men to keep such records, too.

"Why do you want a smear from your rectum if you have no symptoms or complaints?" I asked, avoiding looking at his face with the stubborn goatee. I know these types: they really fancy themselves and their little pleasures.

"Isn't it good policy to check on your health and play safe before anything goes wrong?" he said belligerently.

"There are other ways to play it safe." I volunteered my advice. "Look at this full house. I'm the only doctor today, and I really don't have time to check on your rear. Come tomorrow or next week, or wait till you have some symptoms."

"No," he insisted. "You're here for precisely this purpose."

"You mean I studied for twenty-five years in order to look for no particular reason into your ass?" I was boiling.

But since he did not answer, I proceeded to take the anal smear. He had a special way of bending: turned toward the wall and spreading the cheeks of his buttocks with both hands. The more experienced customers do it like a sort of elegant curtsy or Zen Buddhist bow.

After that I took his blood and thought that I was through with him. But he said very calmly, "And I want a culture of my throat. Last week I had a strep throat."

"That we don't do here," I answered, ready to explode. "We treat only venereal diseases."

"I was told it could be done. I'll write to the Commissioner."

Probably there was something special in the expression of my face when I took him by the arm. He agreed to be led out of the room without any resistance. For the next two hours he sat on a bench, waiting for a social worker or an investigator to register his complaint against me.

155

She was young and cheerful. And huge. Born in Chicago, she attended a school for nurses' aides in Wisconsin (or maybe it was the other way around). Her skin had that particular smooth lilac shade characteristic of the West Indies. There was something fascinating about her: when she undressed she reminded me of a Gauguin painting.

But there was nothing exotic about her gonorrhea, which she acquired from a boy friend who was at nursing school with her.

Later, before leaving, she entered my room again and whispered, familiarly, into my ear: "What's your name, Doctor?"

I told her, adding that I really saw no reason why she had to know.

"But I wanted to thank you properly," she said. "Thank you, Doctor Y." And she shook my hand in the way of women unaccustomed to the gesture.

It was nice enough. A couple of months earlier it would even have elated me, but now I knew better. The strange thing is that when a patient is displeased and imagines himself mistreated, he writes to the Commissioner. When he is satisfied, or even grateful, he simply says so and shakes hands. Thus, in the long run, only *complaints* against the doctor accumulate in the Central Office.

Hate, offense, pride, vengefulness, seem to stimulate more people into writing and acting than gratitude and appreciation. Or do people perhaps expect goodness and efficiency, as if it had been seeded in the universe, and consider malfunctioning an unnatural phenomenon, which they seek to repair?

156

"Where did you get such a whore?" I asked. He was dripping, actually spraying, pus.

"She was feeling sick . . ." he began, "and approached me. . . ."

"What do you mean, sick? Nauseous?"

"Yes, sick to her stomach." He looked at me, surprised by my denseness.

"And then what?"

"She needed her junk. So I gave her six dollars. . . ."

"And she spread her legs?"

"Well, yes . . . She said, 'If you want to enter me, I don't mind. . . .' You know how it is."

Many times I feel like sticking my head out the window and yelling across the boroughs of New York, "No, I don't 'know how it is'! I don't know, and I don't want to know."

157

He arrived with a heavy, helmetlike apparatus over his head and neck.

"What is this?"

"It's a gadget that lets you listen to a program while you are on the move. This way you don't disturb anyone," he explained, flicking a switch on his casket. "Would you like to try it?"

"No, thanks. What's the problem?"

He was discharging from his anus. "I don't seem to be able to get rid of it."

"If you zipped up your ass for a while, that would help!" I said. "What's your job?"

"I'm a psychology teacher."

How absurd. A fellow teaches psychology, wears an expensive device on his head that enables him to listen to a concert or a ball game "while he is on the move," and can't stop copulating for a week. A most peculiar combination: the para-Sodomian elements of a pastoral culture and electronics! Leave him alone on a planet and he will not invent the radio or penicillin, Freudian theory or Einstein's, but his anal activity will apparently continue, supported by horses or dogs if necessary.

158

"When did you last see a woman or a man?"

"This week I've seen only two women."

"How old are you?"

"Seventeen."

"It would be nice if you brought both girls in for treatment."

"I can only bring one. The second I don't know." And as an explanation he added, "You know how it is. . . ."

The next guy who tells me this will get punched in the nose, I promised myself.

159

Since she didn't speak English, I addressed her with one of the few Spanish sentences I've learned: "*Que pasa?*" That surprised her very much, for, underneath her paint, she was Japanese.

"Japanese, Japanese. Ha, ha, ha," or something similar to laughter.

This girl of twenty-two resembled a doll, with the thick layer of lilac paint on her eyelids and her long, needlelike lashes. She was a beautician or, as she called herself, a cosmetician. Her boy friend was a cosmetician, too. He was, right now, on the other side, checking on his V.D. His number was fourteen. It was really amazing how, with only a few words of English at her command, she could furnish all this information.

I went to the other side and spoke to the young man, an American, twenty-eight years old. He had had clap and been treated by a private doctor. He had come along with his girl friend only to make quite sure that he was all right now.

"Come in and ask her whether she is allergic to penicillin. That's the one thing there must be no mistake about."

He came with me to the other side and asked the girl, in English, "Are you allergic to penicillin?" (I could have done that myself.)

She looked at him, expulsed her shy "Ha, ha, ha" laughter, and decided that no, she was not allergic. I took her blood and the smear and gave her two injections for contact gonorrhea. At the critical moments she laughed again, a polite but mirthless laughter, screening her eyes and forehead with her hand.

"How can you understand your boy friend?" I asked. "He doesn't speak Japanese."

"Ha, ha, ha, I understand him," she said.

"Does he understand you?"

"Yes, he understands me. Ha, ha."

"Do you know how you got infected?"

"Yes. Ha, ha."

I was reminded of the Chinese patient from Hong Kong who had watched my every movement without once changing her expression. I felt, at the time, that if I were to use a knife on her she would not bat an eyelash. And now this Japanese "Ha, ha, ha." The future belongs to these peoples. They do not mind pain, and pain is in our future.

122

160

The mother is forty-four; the daughter, who serves as interpreter, twenty. They had come with a letter from the Health Department telling them in Spanish to go immediately to the clinic.

"Why?" I asked.

That they couldn't tell or pretended not to know.

"Is she allergic to penicillin? Did she ever have V.D.? Has she any complaints? Any sores, any rashes?"

Faithfully the daughter transmitted my questions, and the mother, very reluctantly, answered each with a "No."

They walked out of my office, but the daughter immediately returned and told me, "Last month my mother was in the hospital for an operation. Maybe they found something wrong with her blood. She doesn't like to speak to me about it." And without any transition, only breaking into a blissful smile, she said, "I'm getting married next month."

161

"What kind of accent do you have?"

"I'm German."

She explained that she had come to the clinic for a blood test; she had applied for a position as stewardess with Pan American and they demand it. Unfortunately, just last week she went to Puerto Rico for a short vacation. There she met a man who works at the Casino.

"He was so beautiful," she said, smiling euphorically. "But I'm sure he gave me gonorrhea."

"Have you had gonorrhea before?"

"Yes, I have."

"And syphilis?"

"No, not syphilis."

Whatever she said from then on she accompanied with an apologetic smile, as if trying to convey to me that she would make a serious and conscientious stewardess and that this accident in the Casino was an exception.

"He was so beautiful," she kept repeating, firmly believing that that was an excuse even for the Pan Am bosses.

162

A girl who said she was twenty-two, looked seventeen, and needed a bath badly said, "I have a pimple." And she made an almost imperceptible movement with her hips, suggesting that the pimple was somewhere there, between her legs.

I often wonder how they notice these tiny sores inside the vagina. They feel some discomfort there, that is clear. But how are they able to localize it and, even if it has already disappeared, to describe it with precision? It could, of course, be done with the help of a system of mirrors, but I doubt that they take recourse to such means. There must be some special consciousness that men, as a rule, don't have (except homosexuals for their rectum).

163

On my way to the clinic I was stopped in my tracks by the sight of a group of the dancing followers of Krishna. The men with shaved heads, the women with painted foreheads and rings in their nostrils, they were performing a primitive, obsessive dance, jumping up and down, bending and stretching their lean bodies backward and forward, singing monotonously to the beat of an ancient drum their three-

or four-syllable song. All these young American faces seemed joyful, and the fact that they were in constant motion, apparently screaming and dancing for hours without fatigue, was rather miraculous. It might be madness; but since they did not seem to be using drugs or alcohol, this madness, in the center of our dark city, was, on the whole, constructive.

I watched for a while. One of the girls, who was not dancing and singing, moved around the circle of onlookers, talking to them and giving out pamphlets.

"How can she survive such an uninterrupted, convulsive dance?" I asked her, pointing to a member of the team who looked truly possessed.

"It's because she's glorifying Krishna," the girl answered. She looked like a good kid, healthy and sturdy, but in one nostril of her little turned-up nose a hole had been drilled and a ring inserted.

"What are you, Hindu?" I asked.

"No, I was born in England." She smiled a very charming, Western smile.

"Why did you have your nose pierced, stupid girl?" I said. It really hurt me to see the revival of such a barbaric custom.

"My husband likes it," she said, still smiling graciously and ignoring my epithet. "This is a blessing of Krishna. It gives power."

"But why Krishna, why not Christ?" I inquired anxiously.

"Krishna is the father of Christ, stupid!" and, smiling the same smile, she was about to move on. But I felt obliged to do something for Krishna (or for the girl), and I asked for a copy of their illustrated magazine. She gave me one and I handed her a dollar, expecting to get back some change. However, she deftly slipped the dollar into a little leather pouch on her belt and, smiling like a queen, moved on. Apparently it was she who provided for the singing and dancing chorus.

Later, in the clinic, I asked my first customer, a stocky Negro boy, whether he had seen the Krishna followers on the street below.

"Yes, I saw them." He laughed. "I don't object. If you

feel like doing your thing, do it—that's all. If they feel like dancing and singing, they should dance and sing."

"And if, as a result of doing your thing, you end up with sores on the penis, like yours? . . ."

He shook this question off.

"Never mind about the sores. People should do what they feel like doing. Only that way can you find out for yourself."

It was a beautiful morning in May. We should have smelled lilac through the window, but only the monotonous hosannas to Krishna, the new father of Christ, drifted up to us from 125th Street.

> "Hare Krishna Hare Krishna
> Krishna Krishna Hare Hare
> Hare Rama Hare Rama
> Rama Hare Hare Hare"

164

Inscriptions in the john of another clinic:

> My joint is in pain
> Give me something
> To cool me off

(followed by a realistic picture of the "joint")
And underneath:

> Cut the fucking thing off
> You little lamb

(and a drawing of a huge knife)
And:

> Apache and Sugar
> 4 - Ever

165

"What's this?" I pointed to the deep scratches on his arm.

"That's my girl friend. She was playing," he answered, with a condescending smile.

"And she also gave you the drip?"

"No, that was another girl." It was said with cold contempt.

"That one doesn't play, does she?"

"No, she doesn't."

166

Most of our "intellectual" patients are actors, directors, different kinds of assistants connected with the theater, films, photography. They are all unemployed "for the moment," young, and mostly classified S 90, that is, reported as contacts by acutely infected persons. Incidentally, the majority are homosexuals.

This seems to be a closed social stratum, polluted with V.D. (like the waitresses of Old Vienna).

167

"If it's not V.D., what is it? I have a discharge!"

They want to understand. One tries to explain, but most people know more about their cars than about their bodies, and, unfortunately, there are no pamphlets about nonspecific urethritis. What our patients need to understand is that gonorrhea is a urethritis due to gonococci, while nonspecific urethritis is an infection due to a variety of other bacilli that usually are present in our urine. The gonococcal infection we consider a veneral disease; the "nonspecific" infections are not considered venereal and are supposed to be treated at urological clinics.

But to the patients it's all the same—the symptoms are similar and are equally annoying. "What is it? Why am I dripping?" they insist.

My time is limited, and all I can tell them is that if they have a runny nose, it is an infection but not a venereal disease. (By the way, the Russian idiomatic expression for gonorrhea used to be "the hussars' sniffles.") And I advise them to go to the library and look up some books on the subject.

"How come you don't treat me if I have a discharge? The least you can do is explain," insisted the little fellow with the "runny nose."

"I haven't got the time. . . . What are you studying?"

"Shakespeare," he answered with pride.

That gave me a good lead. "All right. Suppose I asked you why Ophelia committed suicide. Would you be able to explain it to me offhand?"

"I think because Hamlet was a homosexual," he told me in perfect good faith.

"Rubbish! She did it because her father, Polonius, fucked her," I explained.

"Oh!" He was genuinely shocked. "I never would have thought of that."

This did the trick: he walked out apparently reconciled to his nonspecific urethritis.

168

"My husband is coming back from overseas. He's in the service. So I thought it would be a good idea to check on V.D. before he arrives. It's the least I can do for him."

"Very nice of you," I agreed, and she nodded, self-satisfied.

As a general rule they expect the doctor to approve any attempt they make to check on their health. They think we are here to protect and prolong their life, regardless of how they have lived in the past and how they intend to conduct themselves in the future.

Penicillin, yes! Morals, no!

169

"How do you feel?"

"Good. I guess I'm cured, although it still burns a little. But I'm worried, Doctor. Three days after you gave me the shot I masturbated. Do you think it could have interfered with the treatment?"

A healthy, pleasant-looking, eighteen-year-old fellow. Naïve? Perhaps a little too naïve. If he did it, why tell me about it? He wants me to repair the possible damage and then he'll go and masturbate again. They seek absolution but reject the priest.

170

A couple: he, nineteen, from Haiti; she, sixteen, a New York Puerto Rican. They are married and both have gonorrhea.

He asked me, "Doctor, how could I have gotten it? I've slept only with my wife."

Her story (later) was: "Before I married I had a boy friend for one year. He was a drug addict. Is it infectious?"

"Is what infectious?"

"Drug addiction. You see, I think I'm pregnant and I want the baby to be healthy." She was a sturdy, very attractive Latin in leather shorts. They call them hot pants, but in this case they were "wet pants." She was really dripping.

"Too much sex," she said. "I'm unemployed and so is my husband and that's all we do."

"You stay in bed together day and night?"

"Yes," she admitted, her childish, madonna-like face expressing genuine sadness. "Too much . . ."

They walked out: she swinging her hips, he with an arm around them, as if, wrapped in those hot, wet pants, was their one and only treasure.

171

A student (probably an exchange student) from Mexico. She had come for a blood test, which is obligatory before admission to the dormitory.

Such a requirement seems logical, but it really makes no sense. The girl may acquire syphilis after she enters school, yet no repeat tests are asked for. Most of the students would profit more from a compulsory bath (with soap!) twice a week; and for the contemporary American woman, a douche would be a revelation.

"Come next week for the result," I told the Mexican. "And if everything is all right, you can get yourself a nice American boy friend."

"Is this a proposition?" she asked, with a sense of humor all the more enchanting because of her foreign accent.

"I wish it was," I answered, and we all laughed, the good laughter of tired people at the end of a working day.

My nurse, a small, boyish, usually beaming Puerto Rican in her early thirties, had been robbed the night before of $400 in cash and a color TV set. Now she laughed for the first time since the burglary.

172

A teacher of Spanish in her early thirties. Single. No complaints, no symptoms, but suddenly she had decided to have a checkup for V.D. "Isn't it a good idea?"

Perhaps it is a good idea—but she hates needles, fears pain, and suffers from vaginism (constricted vagina).

"Don't be rough," she cries hysterically when I try to insert the famous speculum. "What are you, anyway, a butcher?"

"What do you think of Borges?" I try for a diversion.

"Oh, to hell with Borges!" she yells. And at this moment she would say the same about Cervantes, I'm sure. I don't blame her, but if art cannot soften a painful vagina, what is its value?

173

After the twenty-year-old boy had left, a middle-aged, motherly-looking woman came up to me and, in very poor English, tried to find out whether he would soon be all right.

He got his first shot and next week he would get his second, I tried to explain with gestures and words. I thought she was his mother, but later I learned that she was his wife (or mistress).

173

"Over the weekend my girl friend and I were very active. Different things, you know what I mean. . . ."

"No, I don't."

"We sucked and kissed and all that. . . ."

"Yes?"

"Now I have a pimple there." I looked at it.

"It's nothing; it's a simple irritation."

"But why should it hurt?"

This insatiable desire for information, without any personal effort to attain it! They seek pleasure—and afterward they want reassurance.

"Suppose you rowed a boat all Sunday, wouldn't you get calluses?" I tried.

"But I never had it before. Are you sure it's nothing?"

"No, I'm not sure. Come next week for the result of the blood test. Then we'll be sure."

He left, having formed, I felt, a very low opinion of me.

175

"I've come because I think I have gonorrhea and syphilis. My throat hurts and my whole body aches," she told me in a strange basso voice.

"Was your voice always like that, or is it something new?"

"No, it's always like that."

"Have you any sores on your body, any rashes?"

"Yes, I guess so."

She was twenty-two, a student, freshly arrived in New York from Tennessee, two weeks ago. All eyes had followed her when she walked into the clinic with her long, bare legs. But now, on the table, she looked scrawny, pitiful, and inexcusably dirty. Her body was covered with all kinds of sores, which, however, as far as I could judge, were not V.D. Her vagina was full of warts; it was so irritated and painful that I could not insert the speculum.

"They told me I have an inverted uterus," she explained, squirming from pain. "Tell me, is there only one kind of syphilis?" she asked later, in her basso voice, trying to pull her mini-skirt a little lower over her long legs.

They all want to learn something for free, in an easy way. What a wonderful human trait!

"Do you know what a douche is?" I asked, bringing up a subject nearer to my heart.

"Yes. Why? My mother used one. It's red and hangs on the wall."

176

This tiny, slightly crippled woman was sent to us by the court. All court cases are supposed to be examined for V.D.

This morning, she told me, she had put in a Tampax, and now she couldn't take it out.

"Why?"

"I don't know why," she said good-naturedly. "Maybe because I'm so small and the Tampax is so big."

When I tried to locate it, turning my speculum and the light everywhere, I couldn't find it.

"Are you sure you had a Tampax there?" I asked, rather worried.

"Maybe it fell out," she said, with a coquettish wiggle of her body, like a bird or a playful puppy.

She was supposed to be a prostitute, simply a prostitute.

177

A middle-aged black woman, under an enormous, flowery Easter hat the size of an umbrella, brought a letter from her private doctor. He wanted us to give her immediately two shots of penicillin for an old untreated syphilis and to notify him, so that he could sign the certificate she needed for getting married.

178

She is pregnant, in the third month, and has come because her husband is here, being treated for gonorrhea. She had already had a gonorrhea treatment herself four months ago.

"Where does he get these gonorrheas?" I ask.

"I don't know," she says, smiling sadly. Poor little undernourished thing, Gonzales or Pérez by name.

In such cases I feel that we are accomplishing something indisputably good by giving a preventive shot of penicillin (unless, of course, the dose knocks her out).

179

"I'm a homosexual; you have to take the smear from my rectum," he said, looking down at me sternly (he must have been six feet four or five).

"Your friend is a homosexual, too, and I just dug out some gonococci from his front," I said amiably. "A sort of division of labor, what?"

"That's how it is," he explained dogmatically. "One has it in front, the other in the rear."

"If you switched roles for a while, that would give your rectum a chance to recover," I suggested. "And vice versa."

"Yes, it would," he grudgingly agreed.

All dressed, his pants zipped up, he looked, with his bushy mustache, like a pioneer ready to cross the Rocky Mountains.

180

This man, in his late fifties, had had syphilis many years ago and now claimed it had flared up again. And indeed, he had a fresh case, in the typically acute secondary stage, such as we do not see often in New York. (New Yorkers take antibiotics, which distort the manifestations of such infections.)

"Did you pick up someone a month ago?" I asked.

"No, I've been with the same woman for the last six months."

"Only her?"

"Only her!"

"Well, in that case she goofed," I said rather nastily.

He did not answer, this man with the silvery temples which gave him a serene, dignified appearance; with a little luck he could have challenged the incumbent state senator or district attorney.

181

She was a small black girl of seventeen. She came with her son—three years old, a wonderful fellow, who chased me around the clinic, asking again and again whether I was going to give his mother a needle.

His mother was told by her boy friend that she should check for clap.

"And where is the father?"

"The father is away," she answered disgustedly.

"How long has he been away?"

"Three years."

Outside, the boy charged at me again.

"Did you give my mother the needle?"

"Yes, sonny, I did, and if you're a good boy, next time I'll give you a needle, too," I promised.

He smiled angelically and said, "Okay."

182

She was eighteen. Black. Five feet tall. A heroin addict.

"I had a heavy discharge, and my aunt put some medicine in my vagina. My aunt used to be a nurse," she explained.

Her vagina, having been painted with gentian violet, was a solid purple color.

"Oh, a needle. Do I have to have a needle?" she said.

"How come you don't mind all the needles in your arms and legs but you're scared of one needle in your behind?"

She laughed. "It seems goofy, doesn't it?"

"Couldn't you kick your drug habit?" I said. She had such an intelligent (emaciated) face.

"I guess I could. Someday I will."

Nowhere is a miracle so obvious as in the shaking of an addiction. It takes spiritual or intellectual power, and addicts know it. They are aware of the inner forces buried in all of us, upon which they will perhaps draw someday.

Of course there are "scientific" ways of shaking the tobacco or cocaine habit. These are antimiraculous ways, and methadone is one of them. That's why so many addicts instinctively abhor, and are offended by, the very idea of it. For them it means complete surrender of their inner capacities.

183

"My boy friend told me to check on V.D." She was eighteen, with curly blond hair; a bank teller. For some reason we have many female bank tellers with gonorrhea, but no men. (Perhaps the men go to private doctors.)

"Yes, you do have it," I told her a little later. "And a double one, too: in the urethra and in the cervix."

She didn't understand, but she smiled approvingly.

"We'll give you two shots."

"Oh, I hate needles."

"Better tell that to your boy friend. What's his occupation?"

"He's a bus driver."

"A bus driver? Do they have time to run around with girls?" I asked naïvely.

"I wonder, too." She smiled.

"He goofed with another woman. In my time we objected to such things. But your generation doesn't seem to mind," I said.

"My generation minds it, too," she said seriously and sadly.

184

He is sixteen.

"What made you decide to have a checkup?"

"The girl told me to."

"Is she older than you?"

"Yes, two years older."

"Does she go with other boys?"

"Yes, she does, but she's a clean girl. I meant to ask you, is it possible to get clap any other way?"

This question bothers quite a few youngsters. Obviously they would like it better if their partners got it from the toilet or from dishes rather than from sex.

"Lately I've been goofing around with prostitutes, and it occurred to me that I ought to check up on my health."

"Do you have any symptoms, any complaints?"

"No, I have no complaints."

"How long have you been running around with prostitutes?"

"For about three months. I know it's absurd, and I intend to stop."

He was in his late twenties, a white-collar worker, a tense and compulsive type. Who knows why he suddenly decided to go with prostitutes? For him it may have been a heroic act, the first step he ever took on his own.

The other doctor (besides the physician in charge) made it a habit to arrive an hour and a half late. This meant that I processed thirty to thirty-five patients before he appeared, and then we shared the rest. Probably he had some other occupation at the same time, but this didn't suit me and I told him so. He answered that he had nothing to discuss with me. If I wished, I could complain to the Central Office.

I did call up the Central Office, and from there I was advised, "Don't start trouble. He's a Negro. And one of our big shots here is black. You see what I mean?"

I didn't see what he meant, and so I didn't go to that particular clinic any more.

He teaches math at one of the city colleges.

"What's all this information I had to give to the clerk? Is it strictly confidential?"

I glanced at his chart: married, lives in Queens, wife's name Priscilla.

"As far as the doctors are concerned, it's confidential," I said.

"It may be quite embarrassing otherwise."

"Yes, especially with the computers. They collect all the data, and someday, if you get the Nobel Prize or are up for election, they may even blackmail you."

"If I left right now, would you destroy my chart?" he asked briskly.

"Yes," I said, "I'll do it." (I'll do it for Priscilla.)

188

"Ever since I had syphilis I've made it a habit to check on my blood once a year."

"So you've come for your regular blood test, is that it?"

She hesitated for a moment and said, "Yes. Also, the man I was going with last month called me and said he has a blister on his prick."

I looked at her chart: twenty-two years old, treated three years ago for syphilis, and still a weak positive serology.

"Do you have any symptoms, any sores?"

"I had a boil on my buttock, but it's going away."

"How do you know it's a boil?"

"I know a boil when I see one," she answered, with a laugh.

"Can't you stay away from men with blisters on their penises? You're only twenty-two and you've already had your share of V.D."

"I hear it's spreading. They say everybody has it now," she said, seemingly very encouraged by this fact.

189

She could hardly understand my foreign accent. Born in upstate New York, in her early twenties, married, has one child. Her husband had come, too. It was he who had brought her in for a checkup.

"Who gave it to whom?" I asked.

"I don't know," she said. "What difference does it make?"

She wore thick glasses, studied chemistry, and was physically unattractive.

"Why do you live together if you sleep around?" I insisted.

"It's easier that way. It solves a lot of problems."

190

She had come for the third time in three weeks and still hadn't shaken off her gonorrhea.

"How come my boy friend took the pills for two days and got cured? And I had a needle, then capsules, and now again a shot?"

"I don't know," I answered. "We do the best we can. This time I gave you a double dose; maybe it will work. What's your occupation?"

"I'm a librarian."

She was young, frail, and very attractive.

"By the way: no liquor, no spices—"

"And no sex," she finished for me, smiling.

"No sexual stimulation! You understand. No caresses, no petting."

She seemed surprised (they usually are).

"Oh, my! I didn't know that. You see, I haven't had real sex for seven weeks and I'm starved."

191

A blondish female from the West Indies, with a lot of oily white paint on her eyelids. Overdressed, domineering, and looking old for a woman in her thirties. The day before yesterday she went to a city hospital and they gave her tetramycine for her discharge.

"Did you have to pay for the pills?" I asked, noticing the huge vial full of colored capsules she had brought with her.

"No, I'm on Medicaid."

I gave her a shot of penicillin and advised her not to take any more of the pills. Why they gave her 100 capsules is a mystery to me—even if she is on Medicaid. We cure with twenty-four.

192

A twenty-eight-year-old black woman as scrawny as a little girl. She had been in contact with an established syphilitic, and our investigator brought her in.

Instead of admitting her first as an S 90 (which would take the clerk half an hour) and then giving her penicillin and making her wait twenty minutes for a possible reaction, I gave her the shot right away and only then took her chart to the clerk to complete it and "admit" her as an S 90.

When the chart and her personal card came back completed, the bitter, skinny girl could not be found. She had walked out on us. . . .

That's why the old employees don't approve of my treating the patient without delay. But she *did* get her treatment, and I know she'll come back next week!

193

"I'm Alfonso Jesus. Yes, Alfonso Jesus. For Christ's sake, what's going on in New York? I fucked a woman just once, and look. I'm a man with wide experience, and I never saw such pus."

"Why did you fuck such a woman even once?" I asked, always hoping to learn something.

"Why not?" Alfonso was really surprised. "She looked nice and clean." They all use this word "clean," which means much more to them than simple cleanliness.

"How much did you pay?"

"I never pay." He seemed offended. "She came to my apartment as a guest."

He was a jovial, middle-aged man, a kind of Latin gourmand.

194

A child—a small, blond, barefoot child—had been racing through the clinic for a whole hour before I paid attention to it. I thought it was a girl and I said, "This is no place for an innocent little girl!"

"It's a boy," answered the father. "There's no one to take care of him while I'm here."

Daddy—a six-footer in his late twenties, in sandals, slim, with a silky black beard—somewhat resembled Simeon Stylites in one of Buñuel's films. He had come for a trivial gonorrhea.

"The woman I'm seeing now called me and said that she's being treated for clap. So I came, even if I have no symptoms," he explained. The barefoot little boy, sucking his thumb, was standing next to us, listening with no particular interest.

"And where is Mama?" I risked asking.

"She's in New Mexico," Simeon Stylites reported.

"It's filthy here, full of garbage. That child shouldn't be barefoot," I said. "If you had to bring him along, why didn't you put shoes on him?"

"We believe in nature," the father explained.

God save them.

195

"Did you ever have a venereal disease?" I asked him.

"Yes, two or three times," he answered readily.

"What? Syphilis or gonorrhea?"

"Both," he said amiably.

There was nothing extraordinary in the appearance of this thirty-year-old man: rather an average, conservative, positive taxpayer who knows his worth and is satisfied with it.

196

He came in with a paperback: Jacobs . . . something about cities, how to make them beautiful.

He was a personable young man in his middle twenties, with a little pimple on his intimate part and a painful gland in the inguinal region. The Dark Field exposed one pale corkscrewlike *Treponema* epileptically twisting under the cruel beam of light.

Everybody came to look into the microscope. It is always a big catch, and people admire it the way fishermen do when a huge bass or salmon is brought in on the line. I felt that I had achieved something that day, and the doctors around congratulated me with a grain of envy.

"We'll treat you, we'll cure you," I encouraged the pleasant, well-built young man who was shivering with fear. At that moment the future of our cities was the least of his concerns.

197

Sometimes they bring along a guitar, encased in its black sepulcher. I don't know how it starts, whether the young, clap-infected minstrels begin on their own to strum and sing or whether they do it at the urging of the other customers, but more than once I have been interrupted in my work by a concert and have gone out into the waiting room to enjoy the performance. The waiting room is still the same—dark and dingy in spite of all the scrubbing—but the young, hirsute, suddenly inspired faces project a light, a smile, a promise.

Why not have music, poetry, discussions on the meaning of life, love, and art while they are waiting for their smears and blood tests? Perhaps even free coffee? Sort of an agape.

To separate medicine from ethics, philosophy, religion, and art is absurd. We must allow a new form of clinic to come into being, like the new theater, school, or church. But it must come spontaneously. It can't be planned by the Commissioner and his deputies in the Central Office. There must be an openness, a readiness to let it develop, to nurture it wherever it shows itself in the bud.

198

She must "check up on her V.D." Yes, she has reasons for doing it. Age: fourteen years.

A slim, tall child, courageous, with proud eyes. She wears a medallion on her chest: a heavy, round piece, with something similar to a cross sticking out at the six-o'clock position.

"What's this?" I ask.

"Women's Lib," she says belligerently, anticipating ridicule.

"How nice! Is that your girl friend, or is she also a patient?" The two girls had been chatting on the bench in the waiting room.

"No, she isn't a patient. She's my friend."

"You don't belong here," I told her. "You don't have V.D."

She took it as an offense.

199

He had been sent to us by some kind of rehabilitation center. (Rehabilitation usually starts with a checkup for V.D.) I had taken his blood, but he lingered.

"Do you want to talk to me?"

"Yes," said the sixteen-year-old boy, "but may I close the door?"

"Of course. What's bothering you?"

"You see, Doctor," he said, "I have a very small penis, and when I'm with a girl I feel embarrassed. Can it be made to grow?"

"Show it to me!"

He did. "It's not that tiny," I said. "Anyway, I can't help you."

"What I mean, Doctor, is this the average size, or is it small?"

Since he was really anxious I reassured him.

"Average. You have nothing to be ashamed of. Especially if you really like the girl!"

200

A young, voluptuous, but already overweight Negress.

"For the second time this year he drags me here," she complained.

"You mean your husband is here, too?"

"Yes, he's on the men's side."

"How come he fools around when he has such a nice wife?" I asked with real curiosity.

"That's how it is now. It used to be different."

"Do you have children?"

"No."

"What do you use? The pill?"

"No, foam."

"And it works?"

"Yes, it does. But I'm all foam. Everything around me has become foam," she said, looking at me expectantly, as if she hoped that I could solve this riddle for her.

201

Two friends, Oriental-looking, in their late forties, came in together. Both spoke no English, though one understood a little.

"What are you, Chinese or Japanese?"

"We're Korean," he answered, and went on to explain something about a Japanese grandfather.

They both had trouble with their prostates. They made this trouble known by such elaborate gesticulation that some of the patients also understood and laughed. They wanted shots of penicillin. But, since their tests for gonorrhea were negative, I refused, and they continued to chase me through the clinic, showing me very graphically how they suffer when they urinate. One of them claimed that twenty years ago he had been treated for syphilis, so I made him into an S 47 and gave him the appropriate card. The other was offended because he did not get a card of the same kind. He made such a to-do about it that I classified him as a nonspecific urethritis and handed him a card, too. That gave him a right to some pills, and they both retreated, bowing and smiling like actors in a kabuki play.

202

He had a pimple on his scrotum and a painful inguinal gland. A Dark Field was indicated; and, indeed, under the microscope, on the dark background, there appeared the reflection of one pale, exhausted *Spirochaeta*, looking more like a string of pearls than like the usual corkscrew-snake.

The boy—a tall, delicate "intellectual," with a book on some spiritual problems (written by a Frenchman, Paul Lecoeur) under his arm—did not complain throughout the entire procedure and took the news of his illness and the needles with much more fortitude than would many of our "tough" lower-class patients.

147

"Did you examine this patient?" the physician in charge asked.

"Yes, I did."

"How could you miss the sores on the palms of her hands?" The hands were black, the palms were blue, and the blisters were violet. Now I distinguished them.

When she came in I had paid much attention to her past history, fascinated as I was by her wild and sensual air. I asked her whether she had any complaints, any sores on her body, any rashes or ulcers, whether she had ever had venereal disease . . . and all her answers were negative. I looked at her hands and feet, I took the vaginal smear, and I did not notice any pathology.

If it were not for the physician in charge, himself a black, I would have let this whore loose on the streets.

This Negro girl of eighteen put her hand in front of the needle just at the moment when I was about to stick it in her buttock. She got her finger punctured and complained.

She had come to the clinic escorted by a young Negro and pushing a toddler in a stroller.

"Is this your husband?" I asked.

"No, I'm not married."

"Is this your child?"

"Yes," she said.

"And where is Dad?"

"He'll be the daddy." She pointed to her escort.

"Oh!" I felt relieved. "You live together but you're not married."

"No, we don't live together. I live with my mother. I'm pregnant," she explained. All this was rather confusing.

Then came the accident with the needle, and she began to cry like a baby.

205

I saw them coming in only minutes before closing time. She was a plump, young blonde (it turned out that she was in her early thirties, which for us is not so young); he was a giant Negro, carrying a huge, blue crash helmet and other paraphernalia of a motorcyclist.

According to her story, two weeks ago he had caught clap; he came to our clinic, got treatment, and later, after having had intercourse with her, began to drip again. She would like to be checked and treated.

"You mean there is a possibility that you are giving it to him?"

"No, I don't think so," she answered, her blue eyes smiling. "And what difference does it make who gave it to whom? He never came for a checkup after the treatment, did he?"

"That's correct," I agreed. And, plunging the second needle into her muscular buttock, I said, "You're a good sport; you take it on the chin."

"What must be must be. That's my attitude toward life," she said cheerfully.

"What sign are you? What sign of the zodiac?" I asked. (She looked to me like Cancer.)

"I'm Capricorn, the practical one."

"And what's your profession?"

"I am a dancer."

"What kind of dance? Classical ballet?" I tried to suggest something that would sound dignified.

149

"No, just a dancer," she answered, brushing off any further questions.

Indeed, her calves and thighs were strong and muscular.

After the injections I told her, "No sex, no liquor, no spices for a while." She seemed to know that and accepted it easily, but when I added, "And no motorcycling," she was surprised.

"No one ever told me that."

"It irritates the genitourinary system," I explained.

This seemed to make sense to her, and she looked at me with admiration. "What sign are you?" she asked.

"By the way," I said, "what do you do for birth control?"

"Nothing."

"How come? Aren't you afraid of becoming pregnant?"

"No. I had a child ten years ago and since then I've never got pregnant. Something must be wrong inside me."

"Is the child alive?"

"No, he died. Someday I still may have a child." She said it as if trying to console me.

206

"If he lives in Los Angeles, how can you have regular sex with him?"

"It's simple. I'm an airline stewardess and fly there all the time," was her answer. She looked fifteen but was twenty-two—a small, delicate, Oriental creature, apparently born in the United States.

The first tests were negative, but she insisted on treatment.

"He says he has it!" However, when she saw the "big" needles, she drew back.

"What's your idea, did he give it to you or you to him?" I asked to divert her attention.

"Can one get it from kissing?" she asked. "No? Then he gave it to me."

"What's so exciting about kissing?" I said, preparing the second needle.

"Oh, come on! Don't tell me you don't know!" And she laughed triumphantly, like a priestess in her temple.

207

Some girls, particularly South Americans, don't say "boy friend." They use the word "fiancé," thinking that this makes the sexual relationship more acceptable.

Thus, her "fiancé" gave it to her. They planned to get married this month, but now they want to wait till they both are cured.

"How long will the complete treatment take?" she asked.

"A week or two. We'll have to check you again. And where is your fiancé getting his checkup?"

"Oh, he went to a private doctor."

208

He is a strong, good-looking black, apparently with some education and just back from Vietnam. He works at one of the airfields here.

He got it in Vietnam months ago, and can't shake it off in spite of repeated treatments. As soon as he is with a woman the discharge begins again. On and off he takes tablets and capsules a doctor prescribed for him at random. This medication, probably an antibiotic, makes all his smears appear negative, but it does not follow that he is cured. While giving him the injections, I asked him about marijuana in Vietnam.

"Oh," he said, "you can't compare their pot with ours here. There it grows everywhere and everybody smokes it, even children."

"Don't you think it's harmful?"

"Not at all," he said. "I became much more aware and efficient, more dedicated to my work, thanks to marijuana."

"Don't you lose the notion of reality? Isn't time distorted?"

"No. I knew exactly how much time had passed and what hour of the night it was. No, marijuana is completely different from other drugs. It stimulates you for a while, but you're not hooked. No comparison with tobacco. . . . The only bad thing is that it's against the law. One has a guilt complex. If only they would legalize it, there wouldn't be any problem."

I was (and probably still am) against artificial "revelations"; but such a witness—and there are many of them—shakes one's convictions.

209

A very tall black, six feet four or over, in his middle thirties, apparently a workman. He exhibited two chancres on his penis, chancres of such picturesque and classical aspect that I called in several nurses and technicians in order to give them an object lesson. In our age of antibiotics one does not often come across such textbook exhibits.

The huge black, looking much like a great Dane in the small room, first felt embarrassed, but soon began to behave like a movie star or the author of a best seller. He smiled condescendingly and even tried to explain how and at what spot exactly the sore had started. He was especially proud of the fact that he had never felt any pain from the ulcers.

210

A pretty, fair-haired sixteen-year-old girl with a foreign accent. She had come for the results of her blood test. Her bare arms, legs, and throat were silky and china-white.

"What are you, French?"

"No, I'm German," she said, with a provocative and innocent smile.

"Your blood is absolutely all right," I announced, beaming. (The same feeling I used to have when telling a mother after she had come to from the anesthetic: you have a nice girl—or boy.)

"You are okay now," I said. "Go home and don't sin. Or sin only with discrimination."

She smiled, said "Good-bye," and at the door turned back and solemnly added, "And thank you for your advice."

211

He is an airport mechanic.

"Do you service the planes the way they take care of our cars in a garage?" I asked.

"No," he answered. "A car can pull up and stop on the road, and a plane can't."

"Still, I believe any job should be well done," I said rather bitterly.

"They simply have too much work."

"Yes; here in the clinic we also have too many patients!" This observation made him feel uncomfortable. He thought he had contracted syphilis and now expected a thorough examination.

"Doctor, my son drank from my cup. Can he catch it?" he asked anxiously.

"First let's see whether you have it. And, by the way, how about your wife?"

"No, no; she had her period, and so I didn't sleep with her."

Even now menstruation is still a safety valve for the women; except that a way around can be found. Lately, a lot of rectal gonorrhea has been showing up in our literature. That's why the Central Office issued a recommendation to take routinely rectal smears of every woman patient. But we don't follow these instructions. We simply have too much to do.

212

"I don't think it's syphilis," I said.

"What is it, then?"

People like to know. And if we can't figure out an immediate answer we must invent one. This particular young man, apparently an intellectual from a good background, looked pale and worried.

"You said that she bit you, didn't you?"

"Yes." He smiled proudly.

"That's it. A human bite. A chancre does not appear on the penis a day after intercourse."

"But it hurts."

"Yes, it hurts. Maybe it's infected. A human bite is more dangerous than a dog's bite. We are here for V.D., and this isn't V.D."

"You see, Doctor, I already had syphilis once; that's why I'm so worried."

213

One of our clinics has an air conditioner; the others have only fans (and two of our Health Centers have no cooling facilities at all).

The patient comes into my little cubicle, and the first thing he tries to do is close the door. So I say, "Leave the door open for the time being. You don't have to undress right away."

The textbooks say that whatever our patients leave behind, once it has dried out, is not infectious. But the dried-out micromaterial, blown about by the fans, makes us cough. Sometimes we can't shake off this cough for months on end.

214

"What's that? You come every month for a blood test! I don't think it's fair to us. We're understaffed and overworked while you run wild in dark alleys."

It was not very kind of me to speak like that with this very young and obviously insecure fellow, and when he answered I felt ashamed.

"I'm not running wild. After our marriage my wife turned out to have an old syphilis. I was told to check regularly on my blood for a while."

"I'm sorry. I'm really sorry. We have a lot of very inconsiderate patients, and that makes me mad. I'm sorry."

He seemed satisfied with my apologies.

The public-health nurse had just finished indoctrinating a gonorrhea patient. Now she was writing, and the seat in front of her was, for the moment, empty. I sat down and said, "Ma'am, I was told that I have gonorrhea. What is it?"

She laughed—an attractive, tall, middle-aged Negress, very light-skinned, with a classic Spanish profile.

"Sonny," she said, "no spices, no liquor, and no monkey business. *Comprendo?*"

"What do you mean by monkey business?"

"I mean no sex, no petting, no necking, and no masturbation."

"Oh, you cruel thing!" I said. "Tell me, how do they react to such preaching?"

"Some seem to accept it, but most of them laugh. They can't understand it, since they already got their shot of penicillin. The injection is supposed to solve all the problems."

"And what do you tell them?"

"I try to scare them," she said, with a naughty smile.

"Do you tell them that they'll never be cured if they don't behave?"

"No, the old-timers don't believe that. I tell them they won't ever be able to have children." She laughed, quite proud of herself.

"Do they want that much to have children?" This came as a surprise to me.

"Not really. But their ego is hurt. Their manly pride. They want to be almighty. You know—men!"

"What! Don't tell me you're Women's Lib!"

"No, no," she protested. "I like it the way it is. The way it always was. It suits me fine." And she laughed a very fulfilled laughter.

"Miss, I have a secret to tell you," I said in a very official tone. "Your blood test turned out to be positive."

She laughed. "Well, I know someone who will be really worried." The memory of this person seemed to make her happy.

216

After the girl had taken the tests and left my room to wait outside for the results, the nurse who had written up her chart whispered to me, "She's a call girl. How did you like her?"

I didn't like her. Belligerent, incessantly chewing gum, she had spat out her answers like a cornered, poisonous little animal. In addition she was really ugly: small, with acne on her sallow face. She had been traced by our office as a gonorrhea contact, but denied any symptoms and only wanted to know who had given us her name.

When I told her a little later that the test was positive and she had gonorrhea, she suddenly softened and began to cry.

"Why are you crying?" I said. "We'll take care of you. A needle is just a needle. In a week you'll be cured. And if you use your brains you'll never have it again."

"I'm crying," she said, "because I'm worried about my boy friend. He'll have to go through all these tortures, too."

217

When she walked in I had the impression that the Victory of Samothrace was moving toward me in all her power and joy. She wore a sleeveless white blouse and short leather pants. Her long, impeccable, alabaster legs were smooth and cold.

"Do you wear something under your hot pants?" I asked.

"Yes, bikini briefs. Why?" She smiled and looked straight into my mouth as if she wanted to see the words the moment I produced them.

"Just an idea. So what's your problem?"

She had come because her boy friend wanted her to have a checkup. Six months ago she had been in a car accident, and since then she had had troubles with her ovaries.

"Does your boy friend have troubles, too?" I asked.

"Not really. I guess he must be okay. In the police force they look after their men."

When she saw the needle for the blood test, she explained that she had to lie down; otherwise she would faint. I felt disappointed. Some Samothracian Victory!

She lay down on the short gynecological table—pale, cold, and smooth—passed out for a moment (or pretended to, since her pulse stayed strong the whole time), and then recuperated very quickly.

"What's your profession?" I asked.

"I'd like to be a model."

"Don't you want to study something? Learn? Read?"

"Oh," she said, "I never thought of that. That's a good idea."

She was negative on the first tests, but out of esteem for New York's Finest I gave her some antibiotics capsules. ·

She said, "Can my boy friend come here and speak to you? Because he won't believe me that I'm okay. He's crazy."

"If he doesn't trust you, why don't you dump him and find another who will?" I advised her.

"Tell me, are you a physician, a doctor?" she asked, suddenly suspicious.

"What do you think I am, a dentist?"

That made her laugh.

218

She said she was anemic, always on tranquilizers, had had several contacts with suspicious persons (she did not say "men"), and would like to have a V.D. treatment.

"A treatment for what? Syphilis or gonorrhea?" I asked, and added, "It's very rare for lesbians to have gonorrhea."

"I'm not a lesbian," she screeched, ready to throw a fit; but suddenly she changed her mind and continued very reasonably, "I'm not just a lesbian."

She was allergic to penicillin, she said, so I gave her tetracycline capsules as a matter of prevention, even though the test for gonorrhea was negative.

219

A Negro boy, handsome and intelligent (in a Mediterranean way) and without any trace of bitterness or belligerence. No chip on his shoulder!

"I knew immediately I'd be in trouble. I always know."

"How do you know?"

He looked up at the ceiling, trying to mobilize all his youthful mental capacities, and then explained, "When she doesn't smell good, that's my sign."

"If she stinks, why don't you lay off?"

"I see what you mean," he said indulgently, "but it doesn't work that way."

220

He wanted a checkup because he had been in contact with a prostitute. No complaints, no sores, no other symptoms. He looked clean and smart, young and well groomed, so I asked, "How did you happen to go to a prostitute at your age?"

It turned out that during the summer, on weekends, he works in some kind of hotel or lodge in upstate New York. Last weekend a Masonic group came for a vacation: 450 men. They had hired thirty prostitutes from New York City. That's how it happened. And now his girl friend here insisted that he go for a checkup.

"Did you like the prostitute?" I asked.

"Yes, she was really nice. Except that she was worried, always asking me whether I had any V.D."

221

Her boy friend has it. She must have it too. . . . That's how she put it, in her broken English. And indeed, she had it!

"I live with him steady," she said plaintively, "and here I am."

Though I did sympathize with her, I nevertheless tried to make sure she hadn't had contact with other men. That made her think for a long moment and then she asked, "Can you tell me how long it is since I was infected?"

"Why do you ask? So there are other possibilities?"

She smiled a very feminine smile, poisonous and innocent at the same time.

"Yes, there are."

222

"I don't have the urge any more to enter a woman." This he cited as his chief complaint. Forty years old, very stout, with a bulging belly.

"I don't think you belong here," I said, "but we'll make our tests. You should see a psychiatrist."

"What for?" he asked belligerently.

The test showed no gonorrhea.

"If you don't want to see a psychiatrist," I pursued, "go to a G.U. clinic. There may be something wrong with your prostate."

That seemed to tempt him.

"I'll do that," he said, and walked out heavily. He left me with the impression that he had been walking like this from one clinic to another—since eternity.

223

She was only eighteen. The cheeks of her behind looked childlike and innocent. I gave her the 2,400,000-unit dose of penicillin.

"How come your boy friend fools around with other girls?"

"I don't know," she said. "That's what I'm going to ask him."

He, too, had come for treatment and was in the men's wing. A most unprepossessing little fellow, yellowish or jaundiced, who spoke hardly any English. He must have had some qualities to seduce such a sweet girl.

224

"I had a cut on my penis, and now a piece of skin is growing there like a tumor," the boy explained.

"Do you shave your penis?"

"No."

"So how did you cut it?"

"Maybe a girl bit it," he said, with a broad, proud grin.

These biting and scratching girls figure prominently in the life of our adolescents and seem to yield them a special pride (it can hardly be pleasure). Apparently the girls want to leave a conventional mark of possession, a sort of signature, on their temporary partners; and the boys are stupid enough to feel flattered—they think it is a proof of passion.

225

She had long, naked legs. Her face was small, with high cheekbones, and, perhaps because of her eighteen years, it was very attractive. She had already had gonorrhea two years ago; now she was here because her husband had come: he thought he had syphilis.

"I went to visit my folks in upstate New York last week. When I came back, naturally we had sex. Then this bastard tells me that he has a pimple on his private parts," she explained to me. "You know, he acts in those shows where people copulate on the stage. He claims it's only make-believe, but I know better. I forbade him to do it, but while I was away he went back—to get some money."

"And what is your occupation?" I asked.

"Right now, nothing," she said.

It is amazing how many people there are in New York who are doing nothing "right now."

Later I saw her husband. He refused to let the bacteriologist scrape his painful sore for the Dark Field. He looked like an Arab or a Gypsy. How many times I've asked myself what brings such disparate and apparently unequal people together!

"Meanwhile, no sex . . ." I told the girl.

"Of course not," she said, smiling triumphantly as if she knew that she could fool me, her husband, and all men put together.

226

Three young, very young girls came in, joking and laughing—in high spirits! They had all slept with the same man, a musician, and had been told by his steady girl friend that he had V.D. It turned out after the tests that only one of them was positive: gonorrhea of the cervix.

I treated all three to play it safe.

227

Two girls entered my office together. One was already under treatment for syphilis. Being allergic to penicillin, she was taking tetracycline capsules (200 all together) and had come for a fresh supply, since we hand out only forty-eight at a time. The other told me that she had made love with the same boy.

"How come you don't treat me? I had intercourse with him after her."

It made sense—someone in the clinic had goofed—and I quickly gave her a preventive shot of penicillin.

During the examination I said, "In my time we were jealous. We didn't like even our best friends to sleep with our lovers. But you don't seem to mind."

"Why should I mind? I don't care about this boy," she retorted, looking at me as if I had said something very stupid.

"But you slept with him. Doesn't it mean you care?"

"No, it doesn't. When I care about a man I'm jealous."

228

A Puerto Rican woman, a savage-looking young female, with heavy breasts and "no speak English." The investigator told me that her husband, who did speak English, had recently, just before she joined him in New York, acquired syphilis. She should be treated preventively.

"Please don't explain anything to her. I promised her husband she won't be told what it's all about," the investigator pleaded. These poor fellows sometimes have to make the strangest promises so as to get all the parties involved to the clinic.

But the wild female with the heavy breasts, young and very sensuous, looked and smiled as if she understood perfectly well all the implications.

229

"Yes, I have reasons to be worried," the slight seventeen-year-old said. "I made love to a prostitute."

"Oh. And why did you do it?" I asked, seeing that he was really frightened.

"I was crazy, that's why," he explained. Apparently this had been his first attempt to learn directly about sex.

"Did you enjoy it?"

"No, I didn't. The moment I touched her I became panicky."

"How much did it cost you?"

"Twenty-eight dollars. Twenty for her and eight for the room."

230

"I picked up a whore at Fifty-first Street—"

"Fifty-first Street and what Avenue?" I asked, since he had stopped so abruptly.

He looked at me with suspicion but slowly proceeded, "I believe it was Broadway."

"And how much did it cost?"

"I didn't pay."

"I thought you said a whore," I reminded him.

"Well, the way she came with me she must have been a whore."

"And what happened?"

"Nothing special happened," he answered, slightly irritated. "But now I want to check on V.D."

We checked and he turned out negative.

"You see," I said, "maybe she wasn't a whore, after all."

"You never can tell," he answered, very skeptical and very sure of himself.

231

She was nineteen and in her sixth month of pregnancy. She needed a clearance for V.D. to be able to place the baby in a foster home.

"You're not married?" I asked.

"Yes, I am, but we're separated."

"Why did you have to separate at such a critical moment?"

"We are so young," she said. And indeed, she looked pitifully young. "It will do us good to separate and grow up a bit."

"Who will support the child?" I inquired.

"He will, he's a good boy," she explained.

"How long have you been married?"

She thought for a moment and reported, "Almost two years."

232

"Why are you in the House of Correction?" I asked her. She had been sent to us with a letter from that institution.

She laughed.

"They think that I cut up this bitch," she said—a strong, young Negro girl, spreading her powerful legs on the table.

"And did you?"

"No, she cut herself with my knife."

"What was the fight about?"

"She and her pimp jumped my boy friend. So naturally I went after her."

"Is your boy friend in jail, too?"

"No, why should he be?"

233

When they return after a week for the results of the test, and I tell them, "Your blood is all right," they all smile, but they are also shocked and don't know what to do or say next. Some ask, "What now?"

"Go home! You're not sick. You don't belong here."

"Oh! Thank you, thank you!" they repeat with emotion. But somehow they are not convinced.

When I tell them that they have syphilis, they don't thank me. Some even give me a dirty look. But in a way they are more satisfied.

As for me, I am not responsible for the verdict. I am only transmitting a message.

234

A snakelike line stretches from the front door through the hall and down the staircase to the basement. They have all come for smallpox vaccinations: an animated, colorful crowd of laughing and chatting people—middle-aged, youngsters, and even children. They are going to Europe and need a certificate stamped by the Health Department.

At a given point in the hall this crowd crosses with our dismal V.D. customers and then goes its separate way.

What a contrast! Two different universes, touching for a moment and, just as quickly, separating.

235

"Saturday night I went to a party, got drunk, and ended up with a prostitute." That's how he started his story. "Yesterday my wife told me that she has a pimple on her parts. I'd like to check on my blood, because I don't want anything to happen to my wife."

He told me all this quickly and almost in a whisper. A man in his forties, very dried out, with a gray, acne-covered face. Really no beauty. One of those who sit every night in a bar and seem much more interested in their liquor than in the whores around. (I say: seem. . . .)

"You must care a lot about your wife," I observed approvingly.

"I should say so," he confirmed.

"How much did you pay this woman?"

"I don't know. I gave twenty-five dollars to the hotel. . . . I wonder how much she got from it."

236

He was one of those effete-looking, almost pretty stinkers, wearing sandals on his bare, dirty feet and with a heap of music under his arm.

He came in with gonorrhea but, fearing the needles, told me an involved and obscure story of how he fainted the last time he got a shot of penicillin. And yet he didn't have the guts to lie and simply to declare that he was allergic to it. Every time I confronted him with this question he would answer, "No, not really." Finally I marked him "allergic to penicillin" and gave him tetracycline capsules.

A week later he came back with the same gonorrhea, complaining that I hadn't given him penicillin and that I had no right to mark him allergic to it.

We had an unpleasant little exchange, and I gave him two shots. He did perform a sort of collapsing act, but it wasn't an allergic reaction, only a reaction to the pain from the needles.

237

He is an ex-heroin addict, now on methadone. Somewhere they did a blood test, which gave a slightly positive result.

Since heroin addicts very often have a *false* positive reaction, the problem that faces us is to find out whether it is false or true. He furnished no history of previous syphilis, had never noticed any symptoms, and had never had any treatment.

He was twenty-six years old, very tall, very frail—almost emaciated—intelligent-looking, but highly excited.

"How do you like the Methadone Program?" I asked.

"I like it, but they don't give you enough. I'd like to go to a second clinic and get a double dose."

"Does it keep you high?"

"Yes, it does," he said. (I didn't need his answer. It was obvious.)

"But they say it's different. You can perform, keep a job. Is that so?" I asked, trying to get his reaction.

"Yes, it is different," he agreed, without much conviction.

"How many needles did you need when you were on the stuff?"

"From five to ten bags daily."

"That's expensive!"

"Seventy-five bucks." He felt proud of his former daily expense. "But now this blood of mine stops me from getting a good job."

"We'll do a special test that is more precise," I explained. "It takes three weeks, but false responses are much rarer."

"An FTA?" he asked, to my surprise. (That's the Fluorescent Treponemal Antibody-Absorbed test.) Seeing my expression, he continued: "Those of us who are on the Methadone Program, we know everything!"

238

A woman doctor from our clinic, who did her job at least as well as anyone else, was called "fucking bitch" by one of the patients. She retorted: "Get out of here, you fucking whore!"

The whore complained to the Central Office, which, more afraid of public opinion than of anything else, promptly fired the doctor. She made the rounds of the different medical societies, her case was taken up, and, finally, the Central Office had to give in. She was reinstated; but not at the same clinic. She was sent to another borough.

239

He was a middle-aged, muscular black, with the wet eyes and runny nose of an old drug addict. He explained that he had been searched by the police; they had found the capsules of tetramycine that we had given him the day before and had arrested him for unauthorized possession of dangerous drugs. That was his story—and he wanted a certificate from me confirming that he was under treatment.

That the police can be cruel and stupid is no secret to anyone; on the other hand, this fellow could have had some other drugs on him, too. But I did give him the desired statement.

240

A young Negro boy with "killed" veins.

"Do you use heroin?" was my first question.

"I used to, not any more," he answered, with a good smile.

"Are you on methadone?"

"No, God forbid!" He shook his head energetically.

"So how did you get off the hook? Who helped you?"

"My mother," he said, and again smiled his good smile.

"How did she go about it?"

"She talked to me. She took me to the hospital for withdrawal. And then she talked to me some more."

"If only everyone had such a mother," I said.

"Yes," he agreed. And then shook his curly head, as if that would be a complete utopia.

241

"My boy friend gave it to me," she said casually.

She was fifteen, a minor, and her mother had come along with her. She had gonococci in her ureter and cervix (G 11 and G 21).

"I'm not afraid of needles," she announced.

I examined the mother, too, although it seemed absurd. She was clear of any V.D. infection.

"Do you talk to your daughter?"

"Yes, I talk, I talk."

"And it doesn't help?"

"Not much."

"Where is the father?"

"Oh, he's not with us any more."

It turned out that she had two small children at home. So we decided that they, too, should come to be examined for gonorrhea.

She was a lightly colored woman in her early thirties, tall, pleasant-looking, well-groomed, but tired, very tired. A courageous woman with three children, struggling in Harlem.

242

She is from Jamaica. In her late forties. Emaciated, worn-out, but still reflecting her former beauty.

She had recently fractured her hip, and in the hospital they found that "her blood is bad." Indeed, she had syphilis, but her veins were all atrophied from heroin injections.

"Oh, I gave it up many years ago," she assured me. "But the veins didn't come back."

"How did you give it up?" I asked.

"By will power," she said proudly.

She also had cirrhosis of the liver because of alcohol.

"Do you drink a lot?" I asked.

"Not any more. I straightened out."

"How did you do that?"

"I said a prayer," she explained, with the same proud smile.

243

"He's given it to me again."

"Why don't you leave him?"

That she couldn't or wouldn't explain.

"What's your profession?"

"No profession. I take care of my two children."

She was stout, unattractive, twenty-two years old.

"And where's your husband?"

"There is no husband."

We went through a thorough examination, and I said, "Clinically you have syphilis."

"What's that?"

"It's bad blood. It comes from sex with the wrong person."

"Will I get shots? I hate needles," she said.

244

In the course of an examination I do ask rather personal questions. It's hard to draw the line between clinical demands and human curiosity. Sometimes the patient balks, hesitates, or simply won't answer. But I have long since found out that if I hold a pen in my hand and look at the chart, I can ask the most impertinent questions and always get a reply. That is considered objective, scientific, and of possible use in the treatment.

245

Today the three girls from the art school came back for the results of their blood tests. The one whom I had actually treated for gonorrhea wore a new, sleeveless, low-cut summer dress.

They were all negative for syphilis, and they joyfully showed me three diplomas; it turned out that this morning they had graduated from school.

"Well, congratulations!" I said. "Our clinic is certainly the right place to begin an artistic career."

They laughed, and so did two other girls who were sitting on the next bench. They were not patients but friends of the trio and had come along "to keep them company."

"Were you also involved with the same man? With the musician?" I asked them.

First they did not understand my question, then one of the two, a neatly combed Botticelli type in sandals, said, "He means Sidney." And they laughed. "No, we were not involved with Sidney."

Her friend was a statuesque black girl, looking like the Queen of Sheba, in her brightly printed, full-length Indian or African dress.

"What do you think of Sidney?" I asked her.

"I don't think of him," she answered matter-of-factly.

She came from eastern Long Island for the test.

"Can you tell the results to my friend next week, and she'll call me?"

"It's supposed to be private," I explained.

"But it's difficult for me to come in. I don't know how to explain the trips to my parents."

The fact is that, in our crazy life, the Health Department's practice of keeping all information strictly personal often turns out to be cruel and senseless. We force people to come in person; they lose working days or school days, travel, and wait for hours, just to hear whether or not they are all right.

"Will you see the boy again and tell him that he is infected?"

"No, I won't see him."

"How ridiculous, to make love with a person you never want to see again!" I volunteered, and she, instead of brushing me off or calling me a moralistic old fogy from the rotten establishment, agreed.

"Yes, it's disgusting."

She, too, was an art student, and when I asked her whom she liked most among the postimpressionists she answered, "Vuillard."

Bless her soul. None of my previous art students had even heard his name.

"I want you to make all the necessary tests and then to write out a certificate that I have no V.D. . . . . I'm a practical nurse and I know what I'm talking about," she added to convince me. "This bastard went with another woman, and now he blames me for what he got."

"You mean your boy friend has it?" I asked very carefully.

"Yes."

"When did you last have intercourse with him?"

"I never had intercourse with that louse."

"Oh. So how can he accuse you?"

"Because he's a cheater."

"If he's such a cheater, my letter won't convince him, will it?"

She began to cry. She was a tiny, obviously hysterical, black woman of twenty-four.

"Listen," I said, "I have to pass a speculum into your vagina for the test, and I know it's tough for a young woman. Perhaps it's better for you to go home and call it a day before I start?"

"No, I understand, I'll behave," she said, sobbing.

She turned out to be negative all along the line, and that made her happy in a very agitated way. But how it would affect her relationship with the "louse" (who never had intercourse with her) I couldn't figure out.

The investigator, a tall, beautiful blonde of Norwegian extraction, brought in a retarded twenty-year-old girl who had been exposed to syphilis.

"Very nice. But couldn't you bring in your clients before eleven o'clock?" I was angry; ever since nine I had been sitting there, wasting my time, and at the last moment of the session a complicated case was thrust upon me.

Strangely enough, this ugly girl with the crooked nose and dirty hands understood me perfectly and, at first, reacted quite normally. She took the needle for the blood test in good spirits.

Upon examination I found so much filth and infectious material that I could hardly hide my disgust. Clinically she had gonorrhea, and it hurt to think that someone could have abused this little moron. And yet apparently someone had.

Her infected, swollen vagina was so painful that she wouldn't let me touch it with the speculum. I had no choice but to give her penicillin without taking a smear. But now she refused the injection. Every time I touched her skin with the needle she drew away, so that I punctured her several times without having a chance to inject the thick solution. It was already eleven-thirty, and I settled for pills, in the hypocritical hope that she would have enough sense to take them four times a day (altogether there would be 160 capsules!). To let a child like that loose on the streets is a crime; we should be able to hospitalize such cases for a couple of days and treat them adequately.

"Wash your hands!" I told her when she was ready to go. (She had been protecting her inflamed vagina from me.) She very obediently ran to the sink and washed her hands thoroughly, like a good child.

250

They claim that V.D. is rising catastrophically. The Health Department asks for more money, promising a solution of the problem if adequate funds are available. But this is naïve.

During the Great Society of Johnson we had plenty of money, and it did society no good.

The problem of increased V.D. is more complex and more simple than it seems. As long as promiscuity is encouraged and cultivated, V.D. will flourish. Everything around us is increasing disproportionately: cancer, cardiovascular disease, addiction, surgery, crime, welfare recipients. And, of course, communicable diseases. Inflation is the natural law of progress.

People converge on this city because of its liberal social legislation, and they bring with them the plagues of underdeveloped countries, their parasites, and their alien customs. One-third of our patients don't speak English. We get them already formed, with all their obscure backgrounds and festering sores. It's a package deal.

251

There are more than 100 investigators, or V.D. "detectives," in the City of New York. They are supposed to detect and follow up all syphilitics and their contacts. These investigators are ambitious young people who, after a short training, become very important in the system. The police may help them with information and they, in their turn, sometimes co-operate with the police.

There is nothing wrong with helping the police, but this connection between a medical institution and a law-enforcement agency is somewhat unnatural. The investigators become "snoopers." The Central Office, the Health Department, and Albany always get "reports" (most of them clandestine and unofficial) from many sources. Now a certain amount of spying and eavesdropping is taken over by some of the investigators, who, after all, are trained in detective work. As "informants," they become a sort of political police.

Recently, a project to follow up the gonorrhea contacts as well was approved in New York. They got the money for it! That means that now all the sexual contacts of a man during the last two weeks before his visit—and with our customers that usually means several women or men—all those named and identified by the unfortunate lover, must be reached by the investigators. The women are called up at their homes or jobs, visited or written to, and finally (through motivation or fright) brought into the clinic. Here, regardless of the result of the medical examination, they are classified G 90 and given 4,800,000 units of penicillin—unless they claim to be allergic to it. One can imagine what family conflicts and even tragedies are created by this interference in the private lives and the bedrooms of people. Notice that those who can afford to consult a private physician escape all the official reports and investigations and are never asked for their contacts.

Thus, unexpectedly, a most progressive, liberal-minded institution, the Health Department, works at transforming our society into a police state. Personally, if I had to choose between freedom, privacy, and gonorrhea on one side and no freedom, no privacy, and no gonorrhea on the other, I would opt for the first alternative.

252

Whatever the investigators are doing outside, however difficult their tasks in locating contacts, within the clinic, during office hours, they don't work hard. In fact, four or five of them always sit together in their large, clean room, chatting and joking; or they walk to and fro, snooping around.

While our clerks have a hard time coping with the charts, these young people are obviously doing nothing. Three or four doctors may be waiting for one half-literate woman to furnish the chart without which no examination can be started; it would seem natural if the investigators helped the clerks—but no, it's not their responsibility. Besides, the clerks would be offended and confused. Any improvement in the routine "confuses" them, and confusing old employees is considered one of the greatest crimes in any bureaucracy. And the unions don't like it, either.

253

She was twenty-one, looked South American but spoke native New York English. Three months ago she had delivered a child and given it up to an adoption agency.

She had syphilis and gonorrhea, and she was a heroin addict.

"How many injections a day do you need?" I asked, looking at her destroyed veins.

"Four," she answered.

"But that must cost you twenty-four dollars a day!"

"More. Much more," she said condescendingly.

Her boy friend had brought her in: a swarthy man, dressed like a Mediterranean gigolo. He had no V.D. and was not an addict. As her "protector," he asked me many questions, pertinent and impertinent.

"You may also have some gynecological trouble," I told her. "Why don't you go back to the clinic for a checkup?"

He immediately agreed that that was a good idea and said he would take her there.

"Why do you waste yourself?" I asked the girl, point-blank.

She understood me and giggled for an answer. He pretended not to know what I was talking about.

That day the radio told us it was 96° in the shade. Half the doctors were on vacation. The clerks moved slowly, very slowly (we have no air conditioning). But what made the situation desperate was that no bacteriologist had shown up for the session. Without a bacteriologist our clinic might as well close. We tried to proceed by clinical signs alone and, I'm afraid, classified quite a few innocent people as G 10. Then, to soften the blow, we gave them tetracycline capsules instead of penicillin shots.

However, there was no solving the problem of the Dark Field. I told the "suspect" to come back for a special test in the afternoon, hoping that a bacteriologist would be there. This boy from Long Island—blond, pale, depressed—waited for the next session—altogether five hours—obviously without lunch and probably without breakfast. He had an ulcer on his penis that looked like a classic syphilitic chancre.

"Why didn't you come sooner with such an ulcer?" I asked him.

"I couldn't get away to New York, and I couldn't go to a doctor in my town."

In the afternoon we made a Dark Field. It showed one exhausted, anemic, corkscrewlike beast—sufficient to make an immediate diagnosis.

"It's syphilis," I informed the boy from the remote Long Island village. "We'll treat you and we'll cure you. But it's a serious disease. Was this your first sexual experience?"

"No," he said, catching his breath, "I've been with this girl twice."

The waiting-room windows look out onto a schoolyard. In the intervals between patients, while the clerk labors over the next chart, calligraphically printing out names and addresses, I sometimes go to the window and watch the children at play.

Most of our clinics adjoin a local school. Someone had the vision of a saintly Health Department branch in the immediate vicinity of a place of learning: one cultural institution promoting and strengthening the other!

But in reality it is ugly, unnatural. Children in brightly colored clothes scream, swing, slide and race, play ball and turn somersaults next to our V.D. purgatory. In fact, climbing up and clinging to the iron fence, they can—and often do—see the bare buttocks of our patients receive the needles, for most V.D. clinics are on the ground floor.

The children look colorful, but the playground is dismally gray, covered with cement like a prison court, and the jungle gyms remind me of instruments of torture. Why is it all covered with cement? Is it supposed to be hygienic, modern, functional?

I watch the playing children with foreboding. I know that among them are my future clients with the wet pants and the positive Dark Fields. There they are: future muggers, rapists, junkies, racketeers, highjackers, candidates for the electric chair, and, perhaps, a few nominees for the Presidency, Nobel Prize winners, baseball stars, Einsteins.

But usually I think of Sing Sing. The cement, the cages, the dismal lack of greenery, inspire me this way.

"Are you dripping?"

"I was. But may I talk to you first?"

"Make it short; I'm very busy. You can see for yourself."

"Please, Doctor, I came two days ago; you doctors found that I have clap and gave me a shot."

"All right. We'll take another smear to see whether you're cured."

"That's not my question." He began to show signs of impatience. And so did I.

"What *is* the question, man? Speak up!"

He was in his late twenties, short, strong, swarthy, all muscles and tendons—obviously Spanish.

"You see, Doctor, I just came out of prison. Two years they kept me there. I came out and made love only to my wife. . . ."

"Yes . . ."

"How could I have gotten gonorrhea, for Christ's sake?"

"Well, this is a long and complicated story. A very long story . . ." I began slowly to gain time. These family conflicts, especially in the romantic Spanish milieu, don't augur anyone well. "Maybe you had gonorrhea before you went to prison and long ago gave it to your wife."

"That's the point. My wife is here. I want you to find out whether she, too, has it or not," he said, looking at me in a rather frightening way.

On the women's side I found a plump, attractive, though not very clean Spanish woman, with an enigmatic smile and a shocking black eye. Apparently this was the missis. To my surprise her smear was negative. When I told this to her all-muscles-and-tendons husband, he became very agitated.

"I knew it, I knew it, you fucking doctors! You made a mistake. I nearly killed her yesterday. You invented the whole story. I don't have clap, and she doesn't have it. I just came out of prison, where you held me for two fucking years, and now you almost made me kill my wife. I'll sue you, I'll show you fucking bastards what it is to fool around with me!"

In vain did I try to explain to him that there were still more tests to come and that the culture of his wife's discharge would be ready only in two weeks. . . . All he knew was that we were fucking bastards, in cahoots with the fucking establishment, which for some fucking reason had locked him up in a fucking cell.

257

A man in his late forties, small and dried-out, with graying hair; Freud, I guess, would call him an anal sadist. Some years ago he had had syphilis and was cured. What worried him now was that he had been in contact with a boy who, besides syphilis, also had lymphogranuloma venereum.

The boy, a Negro youth, was there, too. He was one of our clients, under treatment for a virulent secondary syphilis. He was covered all over with ashen vesicules, which resembled smallpox. He had come for his second shot of penicillin, but they also expected me to start simultaneous treatment for his lymphogranuloma venereum.

"Look here," I said, "he's toxic, feverish, getting massive treatment for syphilis. Let's wait a week or two, and then we'll give him the other poison, the sulfa drug. Lympho-granuloma is a slowly developing disease; it can wait another week or two." The boy did not participate in our debate, but the "anal sadist" saw it my way, and they left— without the sulfa drug.

Why was this man so intimately connected with that scab-covered youth? Why was he trying so hard to protect him? A new aspect of so-called anal sadism was disclosed to me—a rather sympathetic aspect.

258

He was a dishwasher, and he had come with a skin infection on the dorsum of his hands. It was clear he had severe impetigo and did not belong in a V.D. clinic. So everybody wanted to send him away, to the dermatological department of a city hospital. And yet it was Friday afternoon before the long Fourth of July weekend.

"Impetigo is now easily cured by penicillin. Let's give him a shot, and after the holiday he'll go to a skin clinic. Otherwise he'll lose his job or he'll infect the entire neighborhood around his restaurant," I argued.

"We have no right to do that. It's out of the V.D. jurisdiction," the other doctor, a man with a record of seventeen years in the Health Department, insisted.

I could see that even the nurse in charge was vacillating between common sense and bureaucratic training.

"Suppose he was in contact with a gonorrhea?" I said. "Weren't you lately in contact with a suspicious woman?" I asked the middle-aged Puerto Rican, who was sitting there impassively.

"Sorry, no speak English well," he said, smiling politely.

"You see, he's a typical G 90 and qualifies for a preventive shot of penicillin!" And I gave him the shot.

I felt like the Boy Scout who has done the required good deed for the day.

259

She had come all the way from Texas for a short vacation and ended up in our clinic.

After arriving in New York, she had met her boss from Houston. Of course it had all been prearranged. They had dinner together and then they went to his hotel. She "served him twice," as she put it. Everything was wonderful, although he was no longer young. But now she had a burning sensation when urinating, and there was some discharge.

"Well, we'll take a smear," I told the classic, eternally young secretary.

"Please, make sure," she begged, "because anyway he'll send me to his doctor for a checkup. If I have V.D. he'll get rid of me. He's terribly concerned about his family."

260

He had come to New York for a convention: a middle-aged, middle-sized, middle-earning executive with gray whiskers.

"I noticed a rash on my penis," he said, not sure what tone to take with me, that of boss or of subordinate. The problem was that he didn't want anything to happen to his cherished wife. For himself he "didn't care," he explained. Apparently he considered his private parts as belonging rather to his wife than to himself, and every time he used them it was as if he were spending his wife's savings.

"If you feel this way, why don't you stick to your wife?" I finally asked him.

"I do, but it's not always fun," he answered. "We're middle-aged people, arthritic, short of breath. We know each other too well to really enjoy it. You see, in bed you have to fake, and my wife never fakes. Take, for instance, this whore I was with in the hotel. She made believe so convincingly that she enjoyed me that I was turned on. My wife would laugh," he concluded, half-critically, half-approvingly.

"So whores lie?" I asked.

"Yes." He chuckled. "And that's why you pay them."

"And perhaps liars are whores?" I suggested.

"That I wouldn't say." Suddenly he recovered his executive voice.

261

"The Fourth of July the three of us made love together: another boy, his girl friend, and I. Now I've been told that the boy has gonorrhea. I'd like to check on my rear," said the curly-headed Jewish adolescent, who had come in with a book on chess under his arm.

"The three of you made love simultaneously?" I asked, my ball pen poised.

"Yes," he confirmed, looking hypnotized at the point of the pen.

"And did you enjoy it?"

"Frankly, not," he said with a sigh. "I never had that kind of experience before."

"How old are you?"

"Seventeen."

"And the girl, did she enjoy it?"

"Very much so. At least so she said."

"And the other guy?"

"I don't know, I never saw him again."

"Do you know who Alekhine is?" I continued my investigation.

"No, who is he?"

"You're reading a book about chess and you don't know who Alekhine is? I never was in one of those three-way deals, but I did play chess with Alekhine," I told him vengefully.

262

A youngish man, dressed like an orthodox rabbi, entered. He showed me very discreetly a microscopic pimple on his vermiform penis and demanded on-the-spot assurance that it wasn't syphilis.

"I don't think it is, but the blood analysis will tell for sure. Come back next week." (In my opinion no Dark Field was indicated.)

This didn't satisfy the rabbi. He said he was very worried and would like to know immediately. "If I went to a private doctor, would he be able to tell me right away?" he asked.

"Maybe. You know, money does perform miracles."

But the rabbi didn't smile. He was deadly serious about his pimple.

263

When prospective tourists in need of a smallpox vaccination overflow our premises, some older ones look for a chair to rest on while waiting their turn.

Thus I once found a gray-haired woman and her grandchild, a blond girl of about eleven, on the bench in the men's clinic. The grandmother, tired and short of breath, was obviously suffering from the July heat wave. The girl looked truly angelic: sweet, with clear, light eyes; she was just a hint of a girl, an antinymphet, an anti-Lolita. Both watched my comings and goings attentively but without any trace of embarrassment.

"What are you doing here?" I asked Granny.

"Resting," she answered matter-of-factly. "Anything wrong?"

"No, except that this is a venereal-disease clinic for men."

I had barely a chance to finish my sentence, when Granny, pulling anti-Lolita by her frail, white arm, ran out of the room as if it were on fire. My customers, a dozen or so hairy boys with long sideburns and hussar mustaches, howled with laughter.

I wonder what questions the girl with the clear, light eyes will ask her granny tonight, and what the old crone will choose to tell her.

264

"It seems you had an argument with the male nurse," the physician in charge said. "He complained to the union and they sent an investigator. Now they are all in the Health Officer's office. Come with me."

We went to the third floor and were met by two very efficient-looking Negro women with brief cases.

"He says you called him a stupid bastard," the more intellectual one said.

"No, I believe I called him a stupid ass," I answered, after thinking it over.

"He claims you called him stupid bastard, and there are witnesses."

"I don't think there is much difference between my version and his. This boy is very fresh, really arrogant," and I explained that he tried to run the clinic and tell me what medicines to use.

The intellectual said, "Two wrongs don't make one right. We expect a doctor to show some professional dignity."

"Bullshit," I said politely. "What kind of professional dignity can there be if a nurse or a nurses' aide tells a doctor what to do and what not to do? It's lucky I didn't punch him in the nose. And this stupid guy had the nerve to go and complain!"

It must be stated that the investigators did not press charges. Luckily for me, it turned out that this male nurse had been fresh with others, too, and that they had already had in mind to transfer him back to Harlem.

On my way out, the physician in charge asked me discreetly whether, if the worst came to the worst, I would be willing to apologize.

"Under no circumstances" was my answer.

(For a contrast, see Tchekhov's short story about the doctor who punches his orderly, who then keeps asking for forgiveness.)

265

He looked like St. Nicholas—a young St. Nicholas. A small, bulky man, with an enormous beard joining his uncombed long hair, which was already thinning at the crown of his head. Through this jungle of hair pierced two round, green eyes.

He had just arrived from California for a visit to his mother and had developed a case of gonorrhea—or so it seemed to him.

"Did you hitchhike from California?" I asked.

"Yes, of course."

"It must be easy for you. By now you've probably a perfect technique of hitchhiking."

"It's a simple technique," he said readily. "You must let people know that you are happy and that you wish them happiness."

"By the way," I asked, pointing to his wet underpants, "is this a California strain or a New York State breed?"

He looked at me very candidly, with his round green eyes through the jungle of hair, and slowly, as if making an effort to be truthful, he said, "I really don't know. Isn't it silly?"

266

She was short, no longer young as patients go at our clinics, and, with her crew cut, looked quite repulsive. She had secondary syphilis (papules and macules on the palms of her hands and the soles of her feet); besides, her arms and legs were covered with scars, for she was also a heroin addict.

She had come in the company of a man whom she called "my husband." But when I wanted to insert a speculum into her vagina, she said, "Oh, no, my opening is very small. I must tell you that I don't have sex with men."

"Do you have sex with women?" I asked, momentarily thrown off balance by this disclosure.

She didn't answer. She only smiled—and this sudden smile of hers reflected absolute evil and absolute beauty. Even the nurse was affected by it.

"With whom do you have sex, anyway, with dogs?" she asked.

The patient never spoke a word. Only while I was struggling to find a vein did she say, "Doctor, don't even try. You'll never get a vein from me for taking my blood. It's useless." And again she smiled her beautiful, evil smile.

267

I asked the next patient what book she had been reading while waiting her turn. She showed me the title: *Communication Among Social Bees.*

"Aren't all bees social?" I asked. At that she looked at me with surprise and with all the innocence and attractiveness of a pretty nineteen-year-old girl. "Your tests are negative, you don't have V.D. What made a girl like you come here anyway?"

She smiled a charming, grateful smile. "I lived in a commune, and all the others got it, so I thought I must have it, too," she explained.

"You mean, you all made love to one another?"

"Yes."

"Sort of social bees?"

This time her smile was rather subdued.

"If you continue to have sex without discrimination you are bound to get a venereal disease sooner or later," I said morosely. "Anyway, come back in two weeks for the result of the culture."

"I will. Thank you," she said, and put her hand on my shoulder, a friendly, encouraging gesture, which could be interpreted as an eventual acceptance into the commune.

268

First he wouldn't believe that his blood test did not show syphilis. I had to let him read the report himself. Then he begged me to answer two questions, only two!

"All right," I said, "but only two." (I know how easily two can run into twenty.)

"If I take a test every year and it is always negative, does it mean for sure that I never had syphilis?"

"Yes, that's what it means," I answered without enthusiasm. (If I really knew all those answers I would probably qualify for the Nobel Prize.) By now I was already moving toward the waiting room to call in the next patient. But the neurotic chased after me.

"Tell me, please," he insisted, "why is my urine sometimes purple?"

"Maybe you take some sort of pills," I said, stepping over a chair in order to bypass him.

But he caught up with me.

"Oh! What pills would give such a color?" And he stretched out his hands imploringly toward me.

"Vitamins," I yelled, ducking into the laboratory. "Please speak to this guy," I begged the bacteriologist. "I'm exhausted!"

A long while later I saw them still discussing the color question. The trouble is that we have no time to practice psychiatry.

269

"I've no complaints," she said. "But the man I go out with called and said that he has gonorrhea. The idiot blames me for it."

"And you blame him?"

"No, I don't. He swears he hasn't been with other women, and I believe him."

"Have you seen other men?" I asked the girl, who was plump and very seductive in her scanty summer dress.

"No, not since I've been with him. Is it possible that I got it before and that it never bothered me?"

"Yes, it's possible. There are females who carry it for years without symptoms."

"It doesn't affect them at all?" She seemed fascinated by this idea.

"Eventually it goes deeper, to the ovaries and tubes," I explained. And, although her tests were negative, I added, "Still, let's have a real treatment, since your trustworthy friend claims he got it from you."

She smiled proudly. "I'm sure he *is* trustworthy."

"What's your profession?" I asked. It seemed to me that such a self-assured young woman must have a career.

"I'm a decorator," she answered. "I work for a big house."

"Oh, they are supposed to be all homosexuals," I said, a thought flashing through my mind. "Is your boy friend a homosexual?"

"He was. But he straightened out."

"Straightened out by a crooked woman," I said, smiling broadly to indicate that I was trying to be funny. She laughed, apparently appreciating the joke.

270

"What are you doing here, boy?"

"I'm supposed to get a checkup for syphilis," he explained with a sarcastic wink.

"Why?"

"I don't know. The Youth Center sent me here."

"What are you doing at the Youth Center?" I pursued.

"They are rehabilitating me."

"Rehabilitating from what?"

"I'm a criminal," he said, again winking sarcastically.

"And are you on your way to rehabilitation?"

"Of course, don't you notice it?"

"Did you ever have V.D.?"

"No, never," he said. And I believed him.

He was fourteen years old and did not need a routine

checkup. But bureaucracy is bureaucracy, even in the most benevolent institutions.

271

I walked into the women's waiting room, and from far away a pair of icy, gray-blue eyes, suspended somewhere in the air, looked at me. These eyes, the color of northern lakes in the summer, severe and yet smiling, promised to share their esoteric secret with any man worthy of it.

The girl was twenty-one, of Finnish extraction, silver-blond, and dressed with understated elegance: a long-sleeved silk blouse, a midi-length skirt, and on her head a little cap, like a jockey's, of dark-blue suede, which brought out the color of her eyes and hair. Her story was the usual one: he went to his doctor; he has gonorrhea; he told her to go to the clinic for a checkup.

"What kind of men are these, anyway? They go to a private doctor themselves and send their girls to a public clinic," I said.

The nurse—a tall, heavy, elderly black—did not give the girl a chance to answer. "You better ask what kind of girls these are!" she yelled. "I'd never have such a man. I'd tell him to go fly a kite!"

The girl smiled with her serious, reliable eyes.

"I don't know. I don't see him often enough to talk about things like that," she said.

"What's your profession?" I asked.

"I'm a part-time model."

"That isn't much of a profession. Not for a girl like you," I said.

She smiled to let me know that she appreciated my compliment and immediately turned to practical matters.

"Do I have it or not?"

According to the preliminary tests she didn't.

194

"Should I give you a preventive injection anyhow, or is it perhaps not sure that he has gonorrhea?" I asked.

"You better give me the shot," she said very soberly.

And again her eyes looked as if they had an esoteric secret to share with whoever deserved it. I wonder whether she knew anything about this secret that she was carrying within her.

272

"So he has it and I don't. . . ." She jumped up, a cat ready to scratch, her eyes puncturing me like darts. She was a small, bony, very young, and basically unattractive girl.

"But I'll give you the shot anyhow, for preventive reasons," I explained.

"So I couldn't have given it to him, could I?" she insisted.

"So it seems," I said. "But to be absolutely sure we have to wait for the culture to come back."

"I can't wait; I'm going to Detroit," she said, her eyes burning with revenge.

"Oh, you're going on vacation? That's all right. Come back after your trip."

"I'm not coming back. I live in Detroit. I had my vacation here."

Later I saw the boy friend whose eyes she was ready to scratch out. He was a bulky Greek, with a limited English vocabulary. He seemed very upset.

"Doctor"—he approached me—"can I ask you a question?"

"Yes. One question!"

"How long does it take to find out that you got gonorrhea from a woman?"

"From one day to a week."

"But I slept with two women during the same week," he explained, with difficulty. "How can I figure it out?"

"You can't," I said, impatient by now.

"Can't you tell from the symptoms if it is from the beginning of the week or from the end? Because one of them is my fiancée and I want to marry her."

273

This eighteen-year-old Negro girl, thin, in hot pants, with an Afro hairdo, her features much resembling those of Bette Davis, turned out to have gonorrhea. But when I called for her to give her the shots, there was no answer.

"Don't worry, she's in the park, talking to her boy friend," the nurse said. "She'll be back; I know her kind."

She took one hour to come.

"Did you make peace with your boy friend?" I asked.

"Sort of," she answered, in a dignified and reserved way.

"You aren't angry that he infected you?"

"Why he me? Maybe I infected him," she snapped back, in Women's Lib fashion.

"In my time the man usually gave it to the woman," I explained apologetically. "That is, among decent people."

She smiled condescendingly.

274

An honest-to-God housewife in her middle thirties, screaming hysterically: "I don't care what your tests show! I know I still have it! My husband got rid of it long ago, but I'm still dripping. I want another shot."

She had already gone through several doctors and now had come to me with her complaint, and I finally gave in against my better judgment and ordered an additional injection of penicillin.

"Remember, I won't be able to do it again," I said. "Get hold of yourself. Don't think of it; don't watch it for a couple of weeks. Often it's only psychological. Nerves." (I didn't dare say "neurosis. . . .")

"Oh, thank you, I'll try," she promised, with a good, motherly smile. "You see, Doctor, he doesn't sleep with me because of this discharge. At least, that's his excuse."

275

She is a nice Puerto Rican, who works in the Post Office and refuses the shot of penicillin in her buttocks because she has to stand on her feet all day long. She has come as an S 90: a syphilitic boy, under treatment at our clinic, gave her name and address as a contact.

All her preliminary tests are negative, but in such cases we always give a preventive dose of penicillin—and here she is refusing the shot. What's more, she insists that she never was in real contact with the boy.

"He just sleeps in my apartment because he has no place to go. But we don't make love," she said several times, shyly but with determination. And somehow I believed her.

When I tried to insert the speculum to take a vaginal smear for gonorrhea, she began to laugh hysterically. I desisted and said, "If I give you eighty pills, will you take them—twelve pills a day?"

"Of course," she said.

"Why does he sleep in your apartment?" I asked.

"Because he has no place to go!" she said again. "He's stupid. He'll rot if I throw him out. . . ." Her face shone, with anger (or pity).

276

Some welfare institution had sent him for a checkup. We made a blood test and found it suspicious for syphilis. I ordered an FTA, which is a more accurate but complicated test, and when he rolled up his sleeve the picture became clearer. He was a drug addict! It could very well have been a false positive reaction, important only because it might have dire social (economic) consequences for a patient.

The man was a Negro in his forties, a well-mannered man with a good-natured smile and without any of the bitterness and rebellion to which he was probably entitled.

"I used to do it," he answered to my inquiring look. "I don't any more."

"How did you get off the hook?"

"I got tetanus from a dirty needle and was hospitalized for a year. They did a tracheostomy on me." He pointed to a big, darkish depression on his throat below the Adam's apple. "Oh, it was terrible," and again he smiled his good-natured smile. "I was on a lung machine and a blood pump. Three times my heart stopped, the last time for nine minutes. But when I finally recovered I had lost all urge for the stuff. And now, if my blood's all right, I'll get a job."

"One might say that this terrible disease turned out to be a blessing for you," I remarked.

"How's this?" he asked. "Come again." I explained carefully what I had meant, and this time he understood me.

"Yes," he said with pride, "yes, you can say that again: that terrible disease saved me!"

"I must tell you the whole story," she began.

I mistrust these "whole stories," but she seemed so vulnerable; she was so pale and also so good-looking, and smiled so confidently as she laid her hand on my arm, that I patiently nodded.

She had contracted gonorrhea two years ago in her native state (Colorado), and since then she hadn't been able to shake it off, even after several treatments. She wasn't exactly allergic to penicillin, but after each injection she felt as though her head were going to split open. It so happened she had a mild case of epilepsy; and no doctor ought ever to have given her penicillin. Now she had slept with a man, a very nice man who had called her up afterward to tell her that he had come down with gonorrhea.

"And it's always like that," she said. "I don't want to do it. I know how it'll finish. But they insist. They come at you over and over again, and I can't always refuse, though it doesn't mean much to me."

"How old are you?"

"Twenty."

"And the man?"

"Thirty-four." Here she smiled very maternally.

"Why did you leave Colorado?"

"There are more opportunities in New York. I design dresses, and soon I'll have a collection of my own."

She turned out to be positive on the cervix (G 21) and I said, "Your boy friend is right. Apparently you gave it to him. You'll take these tetracycline pills, and I hope you'll be all right."

She smiled and nodded, as if everybody everywhere said the same thing—always ready to help her.

"Actually I don't have epilepsy," she said thoughtfully.

"I sort of pass out for a second, every so often. I don't notice it, but the others do, and tell me later. And I am a very good cook," she added suddenly.

278

"His girl friend called me up and told me that he has syphilis and that the investigators had asked her to come to the clinic for treatment. So I figured I'd better come, too."

These were the words of an obese, powerful Negro woman, middle-aged-looking, though she was only in her thirties. She seemed excited, and her lips were ashen.

"So you, too, sleep with this man?"

"Occasionally, when he comes to visit our child."

"Oh, I see, you're separated," I said.

"Sort of."

"How old is your child?"

"Which one?" she asked.

That somehow surprised me. "Do you have other children?"

"Yes, I have three from my first husband and one from this fellow."

"You are divorced?"

"I should say so!" she answered.

"Where do you think this fellow picked up his syphilis?"

"What, he?" She shook her powerful shoulders. "Anyplace is good enough for him."

"Could it be from the girl friend who called you?"

"Oh, no. She knows nothing. She's really dumb."

279

She was twenty-eight years old, with pale red hair and pimples on her face. She walked in pushing a stroller, with her boy of two asleep in it.

"Yes, I had syphilis, when I was pregnant." She pointed to the peacefully sleeping boy. "They treated me in the hospital."

But now she had come because her husband was "on the men's side" with a fresh gonorrhea.

"I don't know where he picked it up," she said, with a shrug of her shoulders. And apparently she didn't care, provided we made sure she was free of it.

"But as to your syphilis, you knew where you picked that up?" I asked.

"Yes," she answered, and smiled broadly, her face lighting up. "From him, from my husband, three years ago."

280

This twenty-year-old neurotic walked in with a little sore on his penis. He got it, he said, while making love to a girl; he immediately felt a sharp pain and later noticed the sore.

"I don't know how you could have gotten it; maybe it's just a scratch, but it certainly doesn't look like chancre. To be absolutely sure, come back in a week for the result of the blood test," I told him.

"Are you sure it's not syphilis?"

"I'm as sure as anyone can be about anything in these days in the United States, and now, if you'll excuse me . . ."

"You must think I'm crazy," he persisted, "but I'd like to be sure."

"I don't think you're crazy; I think you're a neurotic. But don't worry, we get neurotics here every day; they all want to be sure."

"Why do you think I'm a neurotic?" His pale face turned yellowish green. "How strange . . . Another doctor told me the same thing. Can it be helped?"

"It's not dangerous; you have nothing to worry about for the moment," I said, patting him on the shoulder and feeling that one more question about his precious person and I'd jump out the window. (Incidentally, this clinic is on the first floor.)

281

"And remember: for one week no sex, no sex at all."

"Oh." She smiled, and for a moment her transparent face became a little more material and opaque. "I can do without it, not only for one week but for two or three."

And she walked out. Very young, proud, almost prissy.

In the hall, a mustachioed, middle-aged man grabbed her by the arm and escorted her to the exit, whispering something in her ear.

Many of them come accompanied by their partners, who have gone before "to their private doctor," and they leave triumphantly, hand in hand, somehow stimulated and happy, as couples leave the maternity ward after delivery.

282

She was tanned all over by the tropical sun.

"Where did you get such a beautiful, even tan?" I asked.

She smiled, flattered.

"In the West Indies. I stayed there for five months with my husband."

"Has he a discharge, too?"

"No, only my boy friends usually get it," she explained matter-of-factly. "It's awful. I make them all miserable."

"All except your husband," I corrected her. "He must be immune."

Again the same flattered smile. "How does it happen?" she inquired. "I feel perfect, and they get infected."

"You are a *femme fatale*," I said.

I don't know whether she understood the expression. By this time her healthy, tanned body was stretched out on the table; naked and taut, it was like that of a strong animal on the defensive.

But here some difficulties developed. Her vagina was filled with a thick contraceptive foam.

"Sorry," I said, "you'll have to clean out this stuff and come again tomorrow for a smear. I can't fight my way through such a mess."

She agreed and we made an appointment for the next day.

Why she had a fresh coat of foam at nine o'clock in the morning was a mystery to me. It was like a soldier carrying a loaded rifle on his furlough.

283

Three women, sent for a checkup: two young girls and one slightly hysterical old prostitute. All three had criminal records and now were sheltered in an institution in order to "kick the stuff"—which means they were heroin addicts.

They came escorted by a sort of matron, a young yet very mature-looking woman, with huge, very white, naked legs.

"How many are there at your place?" I asked her.

"Twenty-nine" was her reluctantly given answer. She was equally reluctant to give precise information about her charges, who were obviously not able to account for themselves. Even when they finally answered my question about penicillin, all three saying "No, not allergic," it remained unconvincing, doubtful. To my question about previous V.D. I received immediately three firm noes, which were just as unconvincing.

"And what about the men?" I asked the matron. "Do they have a separate rehabilitation program?"

"I haven't the foggiest," she answered. "We have no men."

"Aren't you curious to know where men go in such cases?"

"Couldn't care less," she said, looking at me haughtily.

"What are you? Women's Lib?" I asked.

The girls laughed as if I had made a good joke, as if Women's Lib were a very silly invention. But the matron did not laugh, nor did she reply to my question.

There was something queer and cruel in her large, naked, white legs.

284

"So I don't have it and he does." Her eyes glittered like those of a jungle animal.

"Yes, so it seems," I answered. "Now you know what to tell him."

"Say no more." She stopped me short. "May I leave?"

And she walked out: a leopard, a tigress, loose in Manhattan.

285

Our elevator operator had one of her fits today. She stopped the elevator between two floors and began to jump around in the cage, knocking her feet and arms against the wall, screaming, cursing, and rolling her eyes in the most expressive way. She has never done anyone bodily harm, but many of our employees refuse to ride with her and prefer to climb up three floors. That offends her (and may even be responsible for some of her attacks).

The history of this woman is an obscure one, although it is known that for a while she was in a state hospital; whether as patient or elevator operator (or both) remains a moot point. Obviously she is not fit for the job, but it seems that nobody can do anything about this strange situation. When I once spoke to my immediate superior about her, suggesting that she might, through no fault of her own, someday slit someone's throat, I got for an answer that that would be a good opportunity to fire her.

She is a great reader—that is, on normal days. She always has a book with her and speaks to me about literature. She seems very interested in some writers, but her questions are always strange and completely unexpected. Thus she asked me, in connection with Willa Cather's *My Ántonia*, whether it was true that there were many wolves in Russia. On Jung's *Psychological Types*, which, to my surprise, she was reading in the elevator, she asked, "How do doctors distinguish between a big frame, a small frame, and a medium frame in people?"

She wrote out two Russian words from a Tchekhov story and wanted to know their meaning. One was *pud* (an old measure of weight) and the other *muzik* (peasant). When I explained their meaning to her, she remarked angrily, "Something ought to be done about this. They can't simply put foreign words in the text. There ought to be a law against it."

While we had this little discussion, she kept the elevator immobilized between two floors.

She comes every other month: in her late forties, slightly confused, a cowlike, peroxide blonde.

The first few times I still asked her questions.

"Did you have a suspicious companion?" I would say.

"No, I just want to make sure that I'm all right."

"Of course, of course. Are you married?"

"No."

"Single? No man in your life?"

"No man."

"I see."

Her tests are always negative, but I noticed one thing: she usually appears during her period, saturated with blood. Whether this condition especially irritates or stimulates her I don't know, but that is when she shows up. My impression is that she is very lonely, and the visits to the clinic represent a justified entertainment, an ersatz for social and sexual intercourse.

He was sixty-five years old. We seldom see patients of this age in our clinic. In Paris, middle-aged and elderly patients used to be predominant. Many came from the provinces to have a good time with the whores (whom they called *gitanes*, "Gypsies") and then ended up at a consultation at Hôpital Saint-Louis. But here, as a rule, this age group does not indulge. Or, at least, they don't come later to a health clinic.

He had a freshly acquired chancre, and the Dark Field showed us two *Spirochaetae*, dancing as ferociously as mad Gypsies.

The trouble was that he was deaf and could not take in our advice. "Why don't you buy yourself a hearing aid?" I wrote on a piece of paper, after having tried in vain to get through to him.

"I cannot afford it," he wrote back in a very correct old-fashioned hand.

"But a whore he can afford," said the nurse disapprovingly.

288

He was a tall, lean, sweet-looking young man, with very long arms and legs. His elongated face would have served a Modigliani well. He had a little ulcer in his anus, and it was not hemorrhoids—as he had hoped. His Dark Field was positive. (Two positive Dark Fields that morning.)

Before the treatment he asked me, "Could you tell me when about I got infected?" He said it very softly and calmly, while slowly chewing on his gum. I had to raise my head to his lean, long face to catch his words.

"About three weeks ago," I said reluctantly. These precise dates are a pain in the neck. I wonder how the doctors in nineteenth-century novels were always able to predict the exact day when one or another *Dame aux Camélias* would die.

"Yes, that figures," he said calmly. "Three weeks makes sense."

And—young, tall, lean—he froze for my needles, only his jaws slowly continuing the chewing motion.

Young, fair, with white, silky, cool skin, she could have been considered a pretty girl if it weren't for the round ("granny") glasses she was wearing. She was a graduate of a teachers' college.

"What kind of precautions do you take?" I asked. She did not understand my question.

"He means birth control," the nurse explained.

"I've actually had sex only four times," she answered, "three times with rubbers."

"Were those different men or just one?"

"Different men."

After the examination, when she smiled with relief, I asked, "Have you noticed any difference between making love with one man or another?"

"No," she said, "actually I always enjoy it the same. It's fun while it lasts. But later one begins to worry. And these needles for the test actually make you think twice before taking chances again."

Could it be that all graduates of teachers' colleges use the word "actually" so often?

"Actually, I don't see why you came here," I told her. "So far you certainly have nothing to worry about."

"But I intend to come here every time after I've had sex," she said, looking very put out. "Anything wrong with that?"

"Well, well, for once a mature woman," I said.

She gave me the Mediterranean smile, typical of a whorehouse madam, a barmaid, or a temporarily idle card reader.

She complained of burning while urinating.

"Maybe it's the change of life?" she asked coquettishly.

"You claim to be fifty-five. Even that would be a little late for menopause," I said. "What's your sex life like?"

"What the hell!" she exclaimed with pathos. "I'm a widow. I figured that at fifty-five I might as well have as much sex as possible before I go."

"That's right," I said. "Except that some companions are rather unhealthy."

"Don't worry," she said very self-assuredly (cruelly), "I know all about men."

291

"I'll tell you everything," she said, although I hadn't asked for it. "Six months ago I got raped. And since then I haven't been well."

"Did you report it to the police?"

"No, I did not."

"Where did it happen? In the park?"

"No, in my apartment."

"Did you know the person?"

"No."

She was twenty-six years old, divorced (or separated), the mother of two children, and a student of psychology (or sociology). This is Harlem. And, of course, she had an honest-to-goodness case of gonorrhea.

292

This particular nurse happened to be rather pleasant. Deadly inefficient but with good manners. I would say she was a lady's lady.

"You know everything, don't you?" I would drop in passing.

"Yes, everything," she would answer in a snaky hiss.

"And who was Van Gogh?"

"That's not part of my job," she would parry.

One day she really got even with me.

I had just interviewed a woman who looked like a statue: a woman with monumental legs and breasts and a large, round face, framed by an enormous Afro. (Her voice, I did notice, was peculiar, a sort of deep bass, but I paid no further attention to that.) She had come with her boy friend, who was sitting on the bench next to her like a little he-fish.

I sent her to the women's examination room and, when I had a chance, followed her. There I was met by the cobra laughter of the lady's lady.

"Why are you laughing so triumphantly?" I asked.

"I'm laughing at you," she said. "What a fool you made of yourself!"

At that point the physician in charge came up to me and advised me to examine the patient in the men's room. I had seen transvestites before, but never such a perfect one!

"Show me your genitals," I ordered.

"I don't have them right as yet," he-she answered.

"Show me whatever you have."

"She" let down "her" panties, and I saw what seemed to me an empty space below a splendid, bushy mount of Venus. Slowly "it" began to dig lower and finally disengaged a very long, black, silky-soft penis, carefully packed down between the legs (so that originally only a certain elevation was visible).

"You see, they took care of my testicles," he-she explained, "and now they'll construct a vagina." "Her" voice was really striking for a woman.

"Where do you have it done, in which hospital?"

"I go to Europe for that" was the answer.

293

That day, three girls of fourteen or fifteen came in, one after the other. As a rule, our girls are young—younger than the boys. On and off we have a fourteen-year-old male patient, but it is rare.

One of them, a plump, crossed-eyed high-school girl, I remember in particular.

"I have to lie down while you draw my blood, otherwise I'll pass out," she told me.

"Why do you pass out so easily?" I asked.

"I'm a vegetarian, and I'm anemic," she explained, obviously repeating a phrase, her own or someone else's, which she had used many times before.

She had a fulminating gonorrhea, and I couldn't find anything else to ask her but "Why are you a vegetarian?"

"Because I don't want to destroy anything," she said.

"That's very nice. I hope you realize that if you make love to a man with that infection of yours you'll destroy him."

She frowned as if making a supreme effort to understand me, quickly gave up, and, brushing me off with an expressive gesture, said, "I don't know what you're talking about."

294

"Can you tell me how long I've had this disease?" the eighteen-year-old, newly married little girl asked.

"No, I'm afraid I can't tell, although I realize that it would be a big help."

"I'm trying to figure out who gave it to whom," she explained, with an endearing smile.

211

"I understood you from the start, but I can't suggest anything."

She nodded with approval: a plump little housewife who already looked as if she had been married for forty years.

295

This ageless, colorless, sexless Negro man chased after us doctors for nearly two hours. He wanted to ask one question, only one: why can't he perform with a woman?

We couldn't satisfy his curiosity, especially since he had no V.D. and didn't belong in a V.D. clinic. Finally he got hold of a newly hired woman investigator, who shut herself up with the poor fool for quite a while. I don't know what she explained to him, but he seemed pacified and gave up his original idea of complaining to the Central Office.

296

He was six feet two, resplendent with youth and a bright pink shirt. I noticed him in the waiting room, and later, when he entered my office, this impression of brightness and splendor persisted. He smiled at me like an old friend.

"What is it?" I said, casting a glance at the chart. "You're an organist?"

"Yes, I'm an organist."

"Like Bach."

"Yes, like Bach." He laughed.

"What church do you play for?"

He mentioned some Methodist affiliation.

"What's your theology?" Since he looked puzzled, I continued: "Do you have sacraments, communion?"

"Yes, we have communion and baptism."

"To what church is it similar in theology?" I persisted. "To the Calvinists?"

"Yes, I think it's like the Calvinists," he said, without conviction.

No, he has no complaints. But once a year he likes to have a checkup for V.D. "Isn't it a sound idea?"

After I was through with the routine, he said, "You don't practice proctology here, do you?" He had difficulty with the term.

"Proctology? You mean an examination of your anus?"

"Yes, the rear," he conceded, his eyes smiling down on me.

His rear was negative, too, and he walked out triumphantly, his new, pink shirt blazing. I still had a chance to throw him a question: "How's Benjamin Britten? Do you play him?"

"Oh, he's good. We play him a lot," the organist said, with a nod of approval.

297

There are people in their late twenties who already look middle-aged. It seems they won't change any more for the next thirty years. Such was the case of Fred the salesman, who could also have been a bank manager or an administrator in a college or a hospital. His was a "midsummer night's" story. His wife had left with the kids for a two-week vacation, and he got entangled "with a hooker." Now he would like to check on V.D. since his wife was returning the following Sunday.

"You don't have gonorrhea," I said. "As for syphilis, you have to come in a week for the report."

"But, Doctor, you don't understand. My wife is coming the day after tomorrow, and she'll want to make love with me. She always has it on her mind after a vacation. And I don't want to expose her. I love my wife and the kids." He shot

213

me a disapproving look, as if I were the one to endanger his family life.

"When did she have her last period?" I asked.

"Gee, I really don't know. And that's no problem any more. We were told that's the best time; then you can make love without rubbers."

And again he looked at me as if I were the only obstacle to his happiness and well-being.

298

This patient came to me through the men's clinic, although "it" had breasts and exhibited a splendid cleavage. But, painted and perfumed, it had a miserable penis, which dripped pus.

"How come you discharge from the front and not from the rear?" I asked point-blank.

"It" smiled, lowered its beautiful ox eyes, and bashfully whispered, "I don't know how it happened. I've been feeling so depressed lately that nothing made any difference to me."

299

At the end of our conversation the supervisor of nurses shoved her hand under my nose and shouted, "Can't you see this? This!"

Finally I noticed a band with a small diamond on her fourth finger.

"Oh, how nice! Congratulations!" I exclaimed, somehow surprised. We had had so many fights, and during these fights her face and probably mine assumed such ugly expressions that I had never thought of her as a prospective bride.

"I got it last night," she said.

I was about to ask, "Do you know the fellow?" but caught myself in time and said instead, "Have you been going steady with this fellow?"

"Yes, for three years."

"And you plan to get married soon?"

"I guess it won't be long."

"Congratulations!" I repeated; she smiled graciously and ran after another doctor. In fact she was bursting with happiness and wanted to share it with everybody. She's been in this place for fifteen years. But, perhaps, she'll be leaving now. . . .

300

I was parking my car early in the morning, and, while locking the doors, I heard the voice of a bird—a playful, loving voice—expressing some state of happiness. Suddenly I realized that, for a month or so now, the birds had stopped singing: the summer was half over, and the feathered population had settled down to a *petit bourgeois* way of life: raising their young, hunting, quarreling, and cheating to survive.

Yes, summer was almost over, and the birds didn't speak of love any more. This one that treated me to a spring serenade must have been an exception—a bachelor or a dropout. Perhaps a poet?

When I entered the clinic, the huge sign in the middle of the hall greeted me:

And again it struck me that by now all those animated impatient travelers who used to fill up the hall and slowly move in an irregular line down the wide staircase for their obligatory vaccination were far away in the capitals of Europe; that some had already come back, disappointed perhaps, promising themselves that next year they'd do better.

The hall was empty, there was nobody on the stairs, and the idea of vaccinations seemed obsolete.

August had hardly begun, but the summer seemed over. Indeed, some of the tourists were showing up again, but this time not for vaccination. They must have reaped thoroughly in Europe, and now were exhibiting the harvest.

In she breezed, dressed like a troubadour, and yet somehow half-naked. Her tanned back exposed down to the lumbar vertebrae, her smooth skin glowing, her dark eyes glistening. She looked like a young Spaniard of the time of Velázquez, and she even had a hint of a mustache.

"Where were you in Europe?" I asked.

"Oh, I was all over."

"And now you think you have V.D.?"

"Yes, I think so."

"Do you happen to know what strain you got?"

"It must be an English strain," she answered, smiling. "I had sex only in England."

"Did you like it?"

"Like what?"

"Sex in England."

"Well, it's the same, more or less." And she made a movement with her hips as if alluding to some conventional classic dance.

"What are your complaints?" I asked.

"My New York boy friend told me that he has gonorrhea. He thinks I gave it to him."

216

In the second half of August a succession of thunderstorms spanned an entire weekend. Afterward something happened in nature: cool air began to pour in, occasional leaves fluttered to the ground, and the tourists, back from Europe, began to show up in droves at our clinic.

This girl addressed me in a bizarre way: "Love," she said, "listen, love, could you tell me whether I got clap?"

She was tall, with a slight curvature of the spine, and vigorously biting her nails. She was twenty years old, blond and, I dare say, confused.

"I know I have it. I had it before I left, and I took pills for it. But no doctor ever confirmed that I have it. They take my money but they don't make the tests. Incidentally, love, I'm allergic to penicillin." That's how she spoke, occasionally tapping me on the shoulder.

"Where were you in Europe?"

"Different places. Amsterdam."

"Oh, that's the big center for fucking, isn't it?" I said, trying to keep up with her style (perhaps even to be slightly ahead).

"They do believe in free love," she confirmed. "Nothing special, though." Then she continued: "Everybody around me gets gonorrhea. It's so aggravating. I go with a boy and I know the next day he'll blame me for his clap. I'm disappointed in human nature."

"You mean you give it to them?"

"Are you kidding? No doctor ever confirmed it. I take the pills and itch. In Geneva I went to a doctor, a very nice man, no longer young, in his forties. He took a smear and said, 'Jeanne,' he said, 'you don't have gonorrhea. To prove it I'm ready to go to bed with you this minute.' Such a darling, though no longer young. He, too, gave me some pills, just in case. Don't forget, love, I'm allergic to penicillin. Tell me, how do you know that I don't have syphilis?"

She was negative for gonorrhea, and I must admit I, too, gave her pills—just in case. But I did not offer to make love to her. She thanked me, tapped me several times on both shoulders, and told me that she was going off to California the following day—to study art.

"But that makes the blood test I just took absurd; you'll never know the results," I exclaimed, this time really nonplused.

"Yes, it's absurd, isn't it?" She laughed. "Listen, love, I bought some graphics in Switzerland. Do you like Botticelli?" And she handed me a large folder with excellent Botticelli reproductions. For a moment I looked at them, and she, too, over my shoulder, admired Venus rising from the foam.

"That one didn't have V.D.," she said. There was no emotion in her voice. Just a statement.

"No," I said, trying to give her some comfort, "why should she? She *was* Venus."

302

More and more travelers keep returning.

A skinny young woman with a reddish, pelican's nose was telling me about her disappointments in Europe.

"Where did you make love?"

"Only in Italy."

"How did you like Italian men?"

"They're supposed to be great lovers," she said, unconvinced.

"And are they?"

"I wouldn't know. I couldn't compare."

Her nose was really hopeless. I understood why she had to cross the Atlantic to find adventure, she had my sympathy.

303

She came in, all smiles, leaving a trail of perfume behind her. A very attractive brunette, slender, with large, dark eyes. She and her husband had just returned from a tour of Italy. He acquired gonorrhea there, and they both took some pills they bought from a pharmacist in Naples. "Very strong pills," she said.

In fact, her husband wasn't discharging any more, but she wanted to make absolutely sure about herself, since she had heard that it could stay much longer with a woman.

"Did you, too, have an affair in Italy?" I asked.

"No, not this year. Last year I did."

"How do you like Italian men?"

"Very much. They really pay attention to a woman," she said. A little while later the results of the smear came from the lab, and I told her that she still had gonorrhea.

"How strange," she said. "Last year, too, my husband got over it right away and I carried it for months."

"It must be because Italians really appreciate women," I said. She didn't smile.

Both she and her husband were teachers in a New York high school.

304

The patients come in a constant flow. Some have syphilis, some gonorrhea, some have both. But it seems only accidental: if it weren't for a chain of coincidences, they wouldn't be here; they would not have been contaminated.

Then, suddenly, one person walks in and a bell rings in

my ears: Attention! Danger! Watch out! It may be a man, it may be a woman, even an adolescent of either sex, but something unites them: sexually speaking, they are predators.

She looked like a Courrèges model. She was only seventeen, but everything told me that her love cost too much. Be careful! Don't be fooled! Treat her even if she seems all right. Don't let her loose on the streets.

When she exposed her arm I saw from the "tracks" that she was a heroin addict. Disapprovingly I shook my head, and she smiled at me—the sweet smile of an intelligent kitten.

She had come as a contact to an S 30, someone with an old, untreated, latent (not very contagious) syphilis. Normally I could have waited for the results of the blood test without immediate treatment. But in my ears rang this irrational "Danger! Watch out!"

"Can't you join some rehabilitation program?" I asked her.

"I've tried. It takes too long; I never have enough time. When they let me out of prison, before I know it I'm back in again," she explained, and laughed as if making fun of herself.

Preparing my syringe for the preventive treatment, I said, "What's so exciting about heroin?"

"It's not exciting at all. On the contrary, it's relaxing. When it works it relaxes you—no more problems; everything is solved."

"Sort of paradise?"

"It's not paradise. Paradise must be happiness, joy. Here everything disappears—when it works."

"And later?"

"Later, when it doesn't work any more, it's hell," she said thoughtfully.

"So you can get hell but never paradise," I summed up.

She did not answer.

305

A married couple, both heroin addicts. She told me without any question on my part that they wanted to "kick it" and straighten out. "It's never too late to start a new life," she said, and I heartily supported her.

They both had gonorrhea. As for syphilis—we had, of course, trouble to get into a vein.

"Your husband looks like an educated man!" I told the woman by way of encouragement.

"Yes, he is very educated. He teaches retarded children. He's a psychologist," she reported, with obvious pride.

The husband came in with his shoulder pack and right away dropped his pants for the shots, but then immediately pulled them up again and asked, "Is it true that alcohol isn't permitted after penicillin?"

I confirmed that.

He grabbed a half-empty pint of liquor from his bag, lifted it, and was about to drain it, when I stopped him.

"What are you doing?" I yelled.

"I want to finish the bottle first," he explained soberly.

We both glared at each other with more or less the same thought.

"How stupid can a patient be?" was my way of putting it.

"These idiot doctors!" was probably his.

306

She looked like a professional prostitute and was dressed like one. But this was misleading: prostitutes in New York don't look so professional. She came in with a rash on her palms and the soles of her feet, characteristics of secondary syphilis. At eighteen, with her ridiculous beehive of dried-out, peroxided hair, she was pathetic. I found a small pimple just outside the vulva; it seemed tiny and insignificant. Still, I ordered a Dark Field, and this little sore of hers gave us a positive answer.

There is always a sort of jubilation when the microscope reveals on its circular background a dancing *Spirochaeta*, at once hideous and beautiful. We feel jubilant because it is difficult to find it in the field: it has to be the right specimen at the right time, and the search requires a competent bacteriologist.

"Do you know what you have?" I asked the adolescent girl.

"Yes," she said, "secondary syphilis." She must have heard us pronounce those two words.

"How clever you are! Why do you waste yourself? What are you, a high-school dropout?"

"Sort of," she answered.

In general, the answers she gave were vague, foggy: "kind of . . . almost . . . rather . . . possible . . . perhaps . . ."

"You could become a nice person if you went back to school and got a profession," I said, meaning it.

She looked at me with clear, understanding eyes, not the least distorted by the ugly frame of artificial lashes, shadow, and paint.

"Yes, perhaps I will," she said, in the way a mother tells any lie to a child to make him happy.

307

When they walked into the hall I thought the girl couldn't be more than fourteen. Later in my room, facing her, I changed my mind: more likely seventeen.

"I'm twenty," she said, smiling with her big eyes. Her face was emaciated, her body frail and thin, but there was something in her that commanded attention. She reminded me of Botticelli's *Primavera*, especially her hair and her coloring.

"I know I have it because my husband has a discharge," she said.

"Do you know the person who gave it to your husband?"

"It's me who gave it to him," she corrected me, and smiled.

I took her smears. Then her husband came in with a baby in his arms, which he handed over to her. He looked commonplace, with bushy hair and wearing a short-sleeved shirt without a jacket. He was a checker in a supermarket.

"Do you think you have clap?" I asked him.

"Well, it burns, and my wife had an affair recently. So it must be it," he answered very good-naturedly. Heavy and strong, with a large head, he reminded me of an ox.

"Do you, too, have affairs?" I asked.

"Yes, but not so often. I'm tired on the weekend."

While we were waiting for the results of the tests, I approached this family group. The baby looked like an angel in a medieval illumination: long, blond, slightly curly hair, clear, unblinking eyes. Very pale, it smiled abstractedly and did not seem to have much vital force: one of those babies that might be either a boy or a girl and that often die early.

"How old are you, little one?" I asked.

The mother, smiling her Primavera smile, answered, "Seventeen."

"Seventeen months or weeks?"

"Months," she said, with mock reproach.

Father and mother alike were negative for gonorrhea, but I decided to treat them both preventively as contacts. For the blood results they were to return a week later.

She exhibited her poor bony buttocks and held on tightly to the desk while I stuck in the needles and slowly injected the heavy suspension.

"Why do you stay together if you sleep separately?" I asked my eternal question.

"We do sleep together," she said. "I love my husband, and we have a baby to raise."

"Do you believe that's a way to raise a baby? To bring it on and off to our clinic? For it will happen to you again and again."

"But what is there to do?" she asked as fervently as if I possessed some revelation that her mother had not conveyed to her.

"Perhaps you should discriminate a little more."

"But how do you discriminate?" she insisted. "How do you know whether a person has V.D.?"

I didn't feel like telling her to look for sores, wetness, inflammation, and rashes. Instead I said, "You should have some other interests in common with this person. Then, even if you get caught, at least it's worth it."

"You mean not only promiscuity?" She translated my thought with great precision.

The next week all three came for the results of the blood tests. Since she had had penicillin, she felt cured and was dressed in a festive way. In fact, her hairdo seemed to have come right out of the beauty parlor: piled up, shining high on top, and tied with a sky-blue ribbon. It made her resemble a lithe wildcat. No longer Primavera. He looked like a bull, or, rather, like an ox. And the baby resembled the child in Isaiah's vision of the future, when the lion and the lamb will lie down together.

All the tests had come in and were negative.

"What's your name, boy?" I asked the child.

"It's a girl, not a boy," the mother answered in her mock reproachful manner.

"What's your name, girl?"

"Svetlitza," said the mother.

"What kind of name is that?" I was surprised. "Something Slavonic?"

"I invented it," she said, looking expectantly at me.

"Perhaps you should stop inventing and stick to some traditions," I said, unaccountably irate.

She gave me a surprised look, not understanding the reason for my wrath.

308

A little woman of nineteen, good build and good health. Only her colorless, somewhat dull face, with old acne scars, spoiled the impression. She wanted a checkup because last month she was with a man, and ever since she had itched "there."

"What do you use for birth control?"

"Nothing," she said, smiling shyly. "That was the first time I had sex."

"My, my," I could not help exclaiming. "Poor girl, what a disappointment."

"And he couldn't even enter me," she added, expecting further sympathy.

"What, are you still a virgin?"

"Yes, I'm afraid so," and again she smiled her shy smile.

"Your girl friends probably make fun of you," I said, remembering a similar case.

"I don't speak to my girl friends about such things," she said modestly but firmly. It was obvious this little secretary had her principles and convictions.

Since she was a virgin I couldn't insert a speculum to expose the cervix; I took only a vaginal smear (and, of course, a urethral one). The test turned out negative. My impression was that she had trichomoniasis vaginalis, and I told her to see a gynecologist.

"What is that?" she asked, genuinely surprised.

309

"A friend of mine came here from Europe and stayed overnight with me." That's how she presented her story. "And two days later he called up and told me that he has gonorrhea."

"You mean, he thinks that he got it from you?"

"Oh, no, he knows me too well to think such things. Apparently he got it while he was still in Europe."

"What's your nationality?" I asked, expecting to hear Rumanian or Hungarian.

"I lived for eight years in Paris," she said, "but I'm English." (This, somehow, I didn't believe.)

Her test turned out positive for gonorrhea. Sticking the needles into her tender buttocks, I said, "That will teach you not to invite old friends to your house for the night."

"Yes," she agreed, "these days you really can't trust anyone."

310

Her "contact" had a name so complicated that it was easy to remember—perhaps forever. I had treated him the week before, and I asked the fourteen-year-old overweight child, "Are you his girl friend? He was here last week with two other girls."

"I'm his girl friend, too," she announced proudly.

"It doesn't bother you that he has other affairs?"

"No, it doesn't bother me."

"And you, do you also have other friends?"

She took her time and then said, "Yes, I do."

For birth control she was using the pill and had gained twenty pounds in six months. "But now I'm stable."

"Stable and stupid, stable and stupid," I sang, to the tune of a hit song.

311

She was twenty-four, a small, scrawny, unattractive creature.

"I'm a high-school teacher," she told me. "Math."

"And what has brought you here?" I asked, smiling my best smile, intended to calm her, since she was obviously frightened and embarrassed.

"I found out that my fiancé is going with other girls, and I want to make sure that he hasn't passed on one of those terrible diseases to me," she explained in one breath. From her, who had clearly thrown convention to the winds, this obsolete term, "fiancé," surprised me.

Violence as well as fright looked out of her eyes: she wanted her vendetta. She needed one more reason to feel completely free in her hatred for her "fiancé"—and I was to supply it. This final touch would give her the right to hate him irrevocably.

I have noticed that many girls, after a painful separation from their mates, come to us in the secret hope of discovering V.D.

312

"How old are you?" She was sitting in the empty waiting room, a tiny girl with bare legs.

"Twenty."

"And what has brought you here?"

"You see," she began hesitatingly, "my boy friend got gonorrhea, and he told me to have a checkup."

"When did you last have intercourse with him?" I asked rather roughly.

"I don't have intercourse with him."

"You don't?"

"No. We are intimate, but we don't have intercourse."

The word "intimate" introduced order and decency into our conversation.

"Do you have sex with other boys?"

"No." She smiled, forgiving me my naïveté or cynicism.

"You mean you are a virgin?"

"Yes," she confirmed.

"And now you want to check up on V.D. because your boy friend got clap? All right. But please don't tell all this to the clerk. Just say you want a checkup."

She smiled magnanimously with her dark eyes and said, "Of course I won't tell." She behaved as if I were in a comical situation and she wouldn't let me down.

I told the nurse there would be no cervical smear—only a vaginal.

"And why not a cervical?" she asked, her suspicions aroused. (In the public-health clinics the lower echelons are the watchdogs of routine and tradition!)

"She's a virgin," I explained.

"How can she be a virgin and suspect gonorrhea?" The nurse sounded really indignant.

"I don't know, sweetie," I said, "but she is and she does."

It was a hot, muggy day, and the fans bombarded us over and over with the same used-up air (enriched by particles of dried microorganisms). Their noise added to the general feeling of discomfort and confusion.

"What's your occupation?" I asked the pretty virgin, who was negative all the way.

"I want to be a poet," she said, "and write poetry."

313

"You really got it," I said. "Where did you find yourself such a whore?"

"I didn't know she was a whore," the sixteen-year-old answered, looking disillusionedly at his miserable, wet, crushed, sexual organ.

"Where did you pick her up, anyway?" I insisted.

"In school."

"Will you meet her again?"

"I doubt it," he said, surprised.

"How many are you in school?"

"About two thousand," he answered indifferently, still hypnotized by the looks of his penis, watching it as if it were something unfamiliar, alien to him.

314

She was a dried-out, dignified girl of twenty-two, with enormous spectacles; neatly dressed and calm, very, very calm.

"My boy friend and I both had gonorrhea a year ago. We were treated by a private doctor. Now I'm about to go with another man, and I decided to check on my health first."

She had finished and, without any movement or gestures, continued to look straight into my eyes through her huge, round glasses as if wanting to swallow me optically. Very calm and self-controlled, from a good background.

"Oh," I said, "that's decent of you."

She nodded, acknowledging her high moral standards.

"What do you use for birth control?" I asked.

"Nothing, a little foam. I decided that if abortions are

legal and inexpensive, no other complicated measures are necessary."

She was still immobile, without any sign of emotion; her large spectacles reminded me of an animal or insect that I had seen sometime, long ago, in a dream or in an illustrated book (*Alice in Wonderland*, perhaps?).

315

She was crying, the tall, slim girl with shiny chestnut hair and a childish face.

"What happened? Did your boy friend go with another girl?"

"I'm married," she corrected me, very proper despite her tears.

"Has your husband been unfaithful?"

"No, I have." And now she began to sob for real.

She had slept with some man who later told her that he had "a rash." So she came here in agony.

The first test proved negative. "How come you did something like that?" I asked.

"I don't know," she said, still sobbing. "There was a full moon on July fifth."

I glanced at the calendar. July fifth was a Monday, celebrated as the Fourth this year. These long weekends are just as much a curse for us in the V.D. clinics as for the Sanitation Department. There are no statistics establishing the increase of V.D. during the holidays, but it is a fact that people who have no inner life don't know how to use their leisure: they fish or fuck (fuck or play golf).

316

He came in, tall, freshly shaven, in all the glory of his eighteen years. Obviously of good Spanish blood, with a clean, sharp profile; there was something proud and gallant in his manners and speech. My usual customers—hairy, with sideburns, bizarrely dressed—often remind me of the grenadiers of Napoleon's *Grande Armée* during the retreat from Russia. Now they all looked with a certain derision and critical superiority at this neat, well-dressed youth.

I sometimes tell such "outsiders" that they have come too soon to join the old grenadiers, that they should have waited a little, that this is no place for them. And then I'm always reminded of a scene in *War and Peace:* after the victory at Austerlitz, Napoleon rides over the battlefield, enjoying the sight of the numerous dead and wounded. He comes to a group of prisoners—Russian officers of the Guard—and, noticing a very young lieutenant among them, he says, smiling, "*Il est venu bien jeune se frotter à nous.*" "Youth does not prevent one from having courage," replies the officer with a breaking voice. "An excellent answer," acknowledges Napoleon. "Young man, you'll go far."

With different feelings I could say the same thing to many a young patient of mine.

317

Since her chart showed that two years ago she had syphilis and was treated by us, I said, "Apparently you want a new blood test?"

But the twenty-two-year-old blonde with the womanly bosom demurred.

"Let me tell you my story," she insisted. "Some months ago I had an affair—you know, a promiscuous affair." She cast a provocative glance at me. "Usually in such cases it's dark, but this time I left a light on in the bathroom. When I put my mouth on his prick I suddenly saw a red spot. Oh, God, I said to myself, oh, no, not that again! I didn't make an issue out of it, and everything finished fine. But next day I noticed pimples around my mouth. I told him, and he promised to get a checkup. But I never saw him again. Soon after, I met my husband and got married. And now those pimples on my mouth have come back. I'm very worried. . . . If this is syphilis I'll bring my husband here, too."

"Those pimples don't look like V.D.," I explained to her. "Of course, they may come from promiscuity, but they are not syphilis or gonorrhea. In any case, let's wait for the result of the blood test."

She left in a subdued mood, but still carrying triumphantly her promiscuous bosom. That she couldn't help.

318

What a charming little woman! Twenty-two, obviously Spanish: a kitten, a child, a mother, all in one delicate frame. She has been itching for quite a while, and her husband, too, has begun to itch.

"Does your husband go with other women?" I asked. Such a question is not pure curiosity on my part. The answer can indicate possibilities and be of help.

"No," she said, "he has a girl friend, that's all."

"Oh, and do you have a boy friend?"

"No, I'm looking around for something nice," she explained, her dark pupils contracting as if she were seeing someone out of this world approaching her from the other side of the street.

"How long have you been married?"

"Two years. I like my husband. But he doesn't like me."

"Why do you think so?"

"Every time we're in bed he seems to be absent." I nodded sympathetically and she continued, "I guess that's what they call incompatibility."

"You don't have gonorrhea," I told her. "You probably have another infection. It's called trichomoniasis vaginalis. But this is not considered V.D. For that you must go to your gynecologist."

"I have no gynecologist," she told me. "Couldn't you take care of me?"

"No, that's against the rules of the Parks and Recreation Department."

She couldn't appreciate my joke, but she nodded politely.

319

A short stretch of the street is consecrated to doctors' parking. However, all the technicians and investigators park there, too, not to mention trucks and taxis; neighbors and even patients also leave their cars there if they see an empty spot. Thus, the doctors have no room to park. On and off, "brutal" cops descend on this half-block and tow away all the illegally parked cars. One sees breathless, frightened people come running from all directions to save their fifty dollars; it's like an air raid or a sudden small-craft warning.

Since our clinic is next to a tiny park with benches and some conveniently empty ground, I began to park my car there. But one day a fat fellow of retirement age, in a green uniform, came and told me that if I continued to do so he'd have to tow my car away. Those were the rules of the Parks, Recreation and Cultural Affairs Administration.

This little park is a very picturesque place. People from the Bowery come there early in the morning; some perhaps never leave, even at night. They come with all their belongings, with close friends, with food and bottles of liquor. They rest, drink, chat, eat, smoke, and really have a good time, because they are in no hurry whatsoever. A true camaraderie exists among them: they even share their booze and cigarettes.

Facing the entrance of the clinic are two benches, painted purple and orange; there, the companions of our patients wait for them in good weather. Sometimes couples neck there; they don't quite copulate, but apparently the V.D. atmosphere stimulates them and gives them that special sexual kick some people experience in church or in a cemetery. Of course, muggings, rapes, and holdups are also reported from time to time. On different corners of the fence, the Parks, Recreation and Cultural Affairs Administration of the City of New York has nailed its sign:

Enjoy — Run — Hop — Skip — Jump — Litter — Skate — Leap — Laugh — Giggle — Wiggle — Jog — Romp — Swing — Slide — Frolic — Read — Relax — Imbibe — Play — Sleep

The sophisticated trick of this proclamation consists in the fact that on the sign itself all the words underlined above are crossed out with red lines. It seems the Parks Department has its problems, too!

320

I had brought in a black man to the laboratory for the Dark Field. Looking idly through the window, he suddenly realized that New York's Finest were just towing away his double-parked car.

His test was positive for syphilis; and while I was preparing the needles, he watched me with bitterness and pain in his eyes. How much of it could be attributed to the *Spiro-chaetae pallidae* and how much to New York's Finest, I couldn't tell.

321

A bony little creature, with long, lank, blond hair and glasses and with the smile of an irrevocable spinster, came in. She was twenty-two and had been treated by us for gonorrhea two weeks before. I took the repeat smear and told her that according to the microscope she was cured.

The matter seemed settled, but it turned out that the girl who had come along with her was not only her friend but also a potential patient. This one was a sturdy, smiling New Englander of nineteen.

"I don't need a checkup," she protested. "I don't know why she insists. I had all the needles in Germany and France."

"What did you do in Europe?"

"Just touring." By then we were alone, and she continued, still smiling her fresh, innocent smile: "For the last five months I've made love only once. I went to bed with a guy for exactly five minutes. Why should you check on me?"

It appeared from her story that, while visiting her girl friend—that same spinster with the long, lank hair—she was left alone for five minutes with the latter's boy friend and jumped into bed with him.

"Is it nice to make love with your girl friend's boy friend?" I asked this fresh, strong little animal.

"He's hardly her boy friend," she answered with contempt.

She had a good 100 per-cent gonorrhea. When I gave her the shots, she nearly fainted but quickly got hold of herself.

"How strange," she said, "the same thing happened to me in Germany and France. I'm not allergic to penicillin, but I can't stand the pain."

"What did you do in Europe?" I asked again, just to distract her.

"I studied classical guitar," she said, and this answer, under the particular circumstances, sounded so absurd, even to her, that she began to laugh.

The story of the two girls was not yet finished. A little while later I was confronted by the spinster type.

"Doctor," she said, "I'm sure I have clap again. Give me another shot."

"But we treated you and we just checked."

"The boy told me yesterday that he has it," she insisted.

"But the boy was treated together with you two weeks ago," I tried to convince her.

"Not that boy, another boy."

"You know," I said in cold anger, "whores have an excuse: they do it for money. Why do you do it?"

She looked at me, blinking with her colorless eyes and lashes behind the glasses, and said, "Multiple experience."

322

"Apparently you don't understand my problem, Doctor." He looked at me with a shrewd, tribal expression. "My girl friend is coming back from California tomorrow, and you say I should lay off sex. What will I tell her?"

"Tell her the truth if you care about her," I advised. (I was very tired that day.)

He looked at me with the kind of shrewdness that helps men survive in equatorial woods and villages governed by voodoo men, nodded his head, and said, "I see what you mean, but you don't know my girl friend."

"Maybe she, too, had some extracurricular activities in California and would be happy to postpone sex for a while," I volunteered.

"That's their luck," he said, smiling his sophisticated smile. "For a woman it's much easier to invent something about her womb as an excuse. They are wonderful, those women, aren't they?" He seemed full of admiration for womanhood.

323

She wanted to check on V.D. Up to now she had been going only with one man, a married one, but lately she had met a boy whom she liked, so she figured that it might be a good idea to check on her health first.

"Yes, it's a good idea." I supported her without much gusto. "Your initial tests are negative. Come back in two weeks for the rest of them." But she didn't feel like leaving. (An insignificant girl of twenty-two, with claims to be a fashion designer.)

"I want to ask you," she said, "are there any preventive measures besides rubbers?"

"Not that I know of," I said.

"If I stuck only to the married man, would I be safe?" she continued very methodically.

"You can't be sure. That married man may go with other women, too, and besides, his wife can suddenly get some ideas. . . ."

"I see," she said, sparkling brightly with her stupid eyes. "I was told by someone in the know that if you urinate immediately after, you're protected from V.D." She watched intently for my reaction to this revelation.

"Then life would be very easy," I said, gently shoving her to the door. "Everybody would constantly be urinating."

324

A little Puerto Rican with cruel smallpox scars on his ashen, undernourished face.

"I was here last fall," he began, "and now I've come back because I don't want anything to happen again."

"You want to check preventively?" I tried to help him.

"Yes, yes. You see, I was at the movies. And next to me was a girl. You know how it is: we started the usual thing."

"You had intercourse at the movies?" I don't know why I was so shocked.

"Not intercourse. We petted, you know what I mean. And kissed. And now I'm afraid, because I read that you can get it from kissing."

He seemed repulsive to me, but apparently in the dark he represented a symbol: an immense, perhaps infinite image of the male; and that's why an unknown girl, probably also unattractive, felt irresistibly drawn to him.

325

I had a difficult case. An intelligent man who claimed that he never had syphilis but who showed a weak positive reaction in his blood. What should I do? Treat him or repeat the test for possible mistakes? That was my question to the physician in charge. At that moment another dermatologist entered the office, and so I asked this very competent colleague, "What would you do in your private practice with such a patient?"

"Of course I wouldn't treat him on the basis of one serology. I haven't seen a fresh case of syphilis in my office for the last ten years," he answered, surprised by my question.

"But they claim that syphilis is on the rise."

"They lie, as with everything else," he said, with a quiet, sad smile. "It is on the rise as welfare cases are on the rise, as crimes are on the rise. They get a package deal of all these things by letting backward people from poor countries into New York. In private practice you don't see it."

"But gonorrhea is on the rise among the basic population," I insisted, rather shaken.

"I'm not sure. I don't trust their statistics. Among my patients most are repeaters. Anyone who has once had it is likely to come back again. Like criminals to prison."

326

He had come over from Germany a few weeks before. A handsome homosexual in his early twenties. (Some decades ago he could have passed for the ideal Hitler *Jugend* boy: blond, healthy, and obliging.)

"I'm still discharging," he explained, with his polite smile. I gave him an additional shot of penicillin.

When I crossed the waiting room, he asked me, not in the least embarrassed by the presence of all my mustachioed and bearded grenadiers, "Doctor, can it be that I got infected from my dog?"

"What do you mean?" I exclaimed.

"My dog has some kind of infection; he drips from everywhere," he said. "The vet gave him some medicine, but it didn't help. He licks my hands and my toes. Could he have given it to me?"

"I don't think so," I said, still looking at him with suspicion while some of the steady customers shook their heads and rolled up their eyes. "I don't think so. I certainly hope you got it the usual way."

"I hope so, too," he said fervently, and smiled like a naughty boy who has just been forgiven by his teacher.

327

Again I was called to the Health Officer! A public-health nurse (they are a specific breed) had reported my trespasses.

A girl of seventeen, with bare arms and shoulders and in

hot pants, had come for a checkup. She had been there for the same reason five months before. We had taken her smears, and now I went out to the waiting room and told her that the first tests were negative and that she should come back in two weeks for the final results.

"And meanwhile, behave!" I had added.

This, according to the public-health nurse, was a grave error. I shouldn't have said it in front of fifty men and women (who, incidentally, were there for exactly the same reason).

"It's a question of privacy. We must guarantee it to the patients, otherwise they get offended and we might lose our jobs. You know, this is New York," the Health Officer, a sensible, charming woman with a Central European accent, said.

This is New York. A New Yorker takes mugging, raping, holdups, blackouts, transportation failures, rotten mail and telephone service, stupid and/or dishonest car mechanics, criminal judges, corrupted assemblymen, senators, and commissioners in his stride. But such a small breach of privacy a seminaked little girl, a regular customer of a V.D. clinic, cannot swallow. What a fake.

POSTSCRIPTUM

I may as well stop here. If there was a point to be made I must have made it by now.

Some years ago I gave up smoking. I was smoking over three packs a day and felt miserable. Once I caught myself trying to light a cigarette while a half-smoked Camel still dangled from the other corner of my mouth. That gave me the needed shock. I understood that, in reality, I was seeking something else, that tobacco was only a substitute, which obviously did not satisfy me.

I get the same impression now from all these singles, couples, and triangles, young and old, hetero- and homosexuals, these wives, husbands, lovers, and mistresses: they are after something else, and sex is only a substitute, which, apparently, does not satisfy them. It is the job of a teacher, philosopher, or physician to make this clear to every pupil, neighbor, or patient that comes his way.

Every time I stick in my needle I feel: penicillin is not enough!